WITHDRAWN

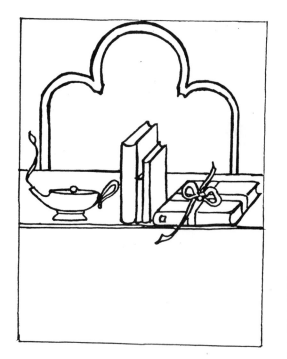

**THE WINSOR SCHOOL
BIRTHDAY BOOK PROGRAM**
Liza Green-Golan '01

5-3-83

DISEASE AND MEDICAL CARE IN THE UNITED STATES

A Medical Atlas of the Twentieth Century

DISEASE AND MEDICAL CARE IN THE UNITED STATES

A Medical Atlas of the Twentieth Century

GARY W. SHANNON

GERALD F. PYLE

MACMILLAN PUBLISHING COMPANY
NEW YORK

Maxwell Macmillan Canada
TORONTO

Maxwell Macmillan International
NEW YORK   OXFORD   SINGAPORE   SYDNEY

Macmillan Publishing Company
866 Third Avenue
New York, NY 10022

Maxwell Macmillan Canada, Inc.
1200 Eglinton Avenue East, Suite 200
Don Mills, Ontario M3C 3N1

Macmillan Publishing Company is part of the
Maxwell Communication Group of Companies

Library of Congress Catalog Card Number: 93–18364

PRINTED IN THE UNITED STATES OF AMERICA

printing number
1 2 3 4 5 6 7 8 9 10

LIBRARY OF CONGRESS CATALOGING-IN-PUBLICATION DATA

Shannon, Gary William.
    Disease and medical care in the United States : a medical atlas of
the twentieth century / Gary W. Shannon, Gerald F. Pyle.
        p. cm.
    Includes bibliographical references and index.
    ISBN 0-02-897371-2 (alk. paper)
    1. Medical geography—United States—Atlases. 2. Epidemiology—
United States—Atlases. I. Pyle, Gerald F. II. Title.
    [DNLM: 1. Morbidity—United States. 2. Mortality—United States.
3. Health Facilities—supply & distribution—United States. WA 900
AA1S5d 1993]
RA804.S54   1993
614.4′273—dc20
DNLM/DLC
for Library of Congress   93–18364
                                                     CIP

Contents

PART III   Medical Care Resources and Treatment Facilities

I

Characteristics of the Population at Risk

1

Historical Overview

It is important to document a nation's historical experience with health, disease, death, and medical care. The resulting data reflect the evolution of many dimensions of society. Over the course of the twentieth century—through economic development; improvements in housing and sanitation; implementation of public health programs to prevent and control certain diseases; and development of improved medical technology for diagnosing, assessing, and treating medical problems—both the characteristics and the life and death experience of the population of the United States have been dramatically altered. As in the past, however, the nation's experience is not uniform; considerable variation exists from state to state in each dimension of the experience. It is the authors' belief that by describing and illustrating the differences between states we can contribute to a better understanding of the complex mosaic which is the United States. In this volume we hope to demonstrate some of the differences and their significance.

Population Changes

As mentioned above, important changes in the population characteristics of the United States have taken place during the twentieth century. In 1900 the total population of the United States was just over 76 million people. By 1990, the population had more than tripled, to over 250 million people. The total 1900 population of the United States is today equaled by the combined populations of only four large states: California, New York, Texas, and Pennsylvania. The U.S. population is projected to increase to an estimated 270 million by the year 2000. While a substantial proportion of this population growth is due to immigration, a large part is also due to changes in the rate of natural increase, that is, to the relationship between birth rates and death rates.

People are living longer today. The average life expectancy for a child born in the United States in 1900 was about 47 years—46 years for males and 48 years for females. By contrast the average life expectancy for a child born in 1991 exceeds 75 years—almost 72 years for males and over 78 years for females. Moreover, on average, a person who was 65 years old in 1900 could expect to live an additional 12 years. Today the average life expectancy of a 65-year-old person is over 17 years—about 15 years for males and 19 years for females.

Deaths and Diseases

More children are also surviving the crucial first year of life today than in the past. Today, on average, for every 1,000 live births fewer than 10 children die before their first birthdays. While this may seem a high figure, it is lower by a factor of 10 than the estimated infant mortality rate of well over 100 for every 1,000 live births at the turn of the century.

Just as there has been a decrease in infant mortality, there has also been a gradual decrease in the overall death rate in the United States. In 1900 more than 17 people out of every 1,000 people in the United States died. In contrast, the most recent data indicate that the annual death rate has been reduced to about 5 people out of every 1,000.

The major causes of death have also changed substantially. Diseases which were once major killers have now been reduced to minor roles, while other diseases and conditions have taken their place as major threats to health. Tuberculosis and pneumonia were the leading killers in 1900. Almost 200 of every 100,000 deaths in 1900 were caused by tuberculosis; today tuberculosis in all its forms accounts for fewer than 1 death in 100,000. An additional 200 of every 100,000 deaths resulted from pneumonia. In addition, substantial numbers of deaths were attributed to diarrheal diseases, diptheria, typhoid fever, bronchitis, and even cholera. Many of the causes of death in 1900 have been substantially reduced in importance, some to virtual insignificance today. Others have retained or even increased their significance. While heart disease in all its forms was among the leading killers in 1900, today it is the primary cause of death, followed by cancer, cerebrovascular disease, and accidents.

Most diseases are continuously circulating through the population. From time to time, however, old or new diseases emerge or occur in acute epidemic form. This phenomenon severely affects morbidity and mortality patterns in the United States. In 1918, for example, the population of the United States was hard hit by a pandemic (worldwide epidemic) of influenza, the worst in recorded history. In the winter of 1918–1919, more than 500,000 people in the United States died of influenza and its complications. In a more recent development, which is not as acute and not yet as devastating, since 1981 over 170,000 persons in the United States have died of diseases and conditions associated with what is believed to be a new form of disease, the acquired immune deficiency syndrome (AIDS). To date there is no cure for this fatal infectious disease, and the future course of this pandemic has yet to be accurately charted for the United States and the world.

Apart from diseases, other factors that pose significant threats to health have developed in the United States. The twentieth century has witnessed the rise of the automobile to dominance, and the consequential modification of United States society in many ways. The proliferation of the automobile has had and continues to have serious consequences, which pose both direct and indirect threats to health. Certainly, the pollutants emitted in exhaust from combustible engines have contributed to a deterioration of the atmosphere and increased the number of health problems and deaths in the United States. More directly, the number of traffic-related deaths per year, which was not even listed in 1900, has risen to over 50,000. The number of persons who receive nonfatal injuries in automobile accidents is over 3.5 million annually. The automobile represents both a way of life and a significant threat to health and life for most people. Among certain groups, particularly males 16 to 24 years old, the automobile is the major threat to life.

The Death Registration Area

The annual collection of mortality statistics by the Bureau of the Census began with the calendar year 1900. The statistics were not collected from all the states, however. In effect, states had to qualify to be included in the developing national Death Registration Area, (the official name for the emerging national system). To be included in the system, a state had to have a minimum of 90 percent of deaths regularly registered and was also required to adopt a standard death certificate by January 1, 1900. Only 10 states, plus the District of Columbia (which was included as a state), and 153 registration cities located in nonregistration states were included in the initial Death Registration Area (Figure 1.1). To qualify, as a distinct geographical unit, cities had to have a minimum of 8,000 residents, and the registration of deaths under local laws and ordinances had to be sufficiently accurate for use by the Census Office. Though the cities were widely distributed, the initial group of states was located predominantly in the Northeast. These states and cities were estimated to include about 38 percent of the entire population in 1900. Periodically, additional states qualified to be included in the Death Registration Area. Occasionally, a state (Delaware, South Dakota, and Georgia are examples) would fail to maintain the necessary standards of reporting and would be temporarily dropped from the list. By 1910, the Death Registration Area included 21 states and the District of Columbia. More states were added, and the addition of Nebraska in 1920 brought the total to 34. With the inclusion of Texas in 1933, the national system of reporting was complete; it included all 48 states. Alaska was added upon its admission in 1959. Hawaii, admitted later in the same year, was added to the Death Registration Area in 1960.

The changing composition of the Death Registration Area is important because it was impossible to obtain geographically comparable state mortality data for the entire nation prior to 1933. Nevertheless, the published rates based on this expanding group of registration states and cities do approximate national rates over the period, and general comparisons over long periods are made in this book.

Medical Care

A number of factors, some known and many more unknown, contribute to changes in vulnerability to dis-

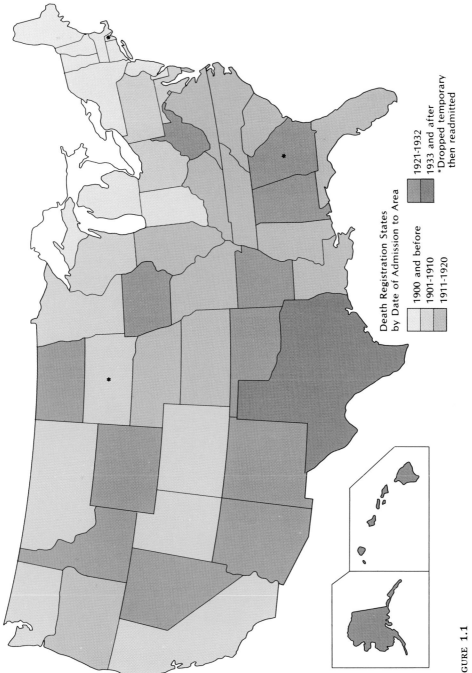

Death Registration States
by Date of Admission to Area

1900 and before
1901-1910
1911-1920
1921-1932
1933 and after
*Dropped temporary
then readmitted

FIGURE 1.1
Development of National Death Registration Area

5

ease and death. Improvements in sanitation, nutrition, and housing during this century have contributed substantially to a longer-lived and healthier, population. Major public health programs of immunization and preventive health care have significantly reduced the threats of some specific diseases, especially those which occur most frequently among children. Certain treatments have extended the lives of many elderly people. While debate continues about the relative significance of the medical care sector, including hospitals and physicians, for individual health, the population as a whole are undoubtedly dependent upon them in times of sickness or injury.

The Use of Hospitals

In the late nineteenth and early twentieth centuries, hospitals were shunned by everyone but the very poor. A radical transformation has occurred: for most people today hospitals represent the use of surgical intervention and specialized medical care and research. Perhaps because of an inability to determine the appropriate number and distribution of hospital beds for a given population, the history of hospital growth has been variable. Periods of rapid expansion have been intermingled with periods of stagnation and even decline. In 1909 there were approximately 4,300 community hospitals in the United States, containing just over 400,000 beds. There are now about 5,500 short-term registered non-federal- and non-state-supported community hospitals in the United States, with a little less than one million beds.

Within the hospital sector the most significant changes have come about in terms of long-term hospital facilities for the mentally ill. From 1900 through 1955 there was a steady increase in the number of hospital beds in state-supported asylums or hospitals for the mentally ill. By 1955, over 500,000 patients resided in these facilities. The confluence of a number of developments in the philosophy and treatment regimen of the mentally ill subsequently led to a wholesale dismantling of the mental hospital system and to deinstitutionalization of many mentally ill people. The number of state-supported long-term hospital beds for the mentally ill and the number of patients in these facilities has fallen to about 100,000. Today this process is considered by many to be a mistake.

The Role of the Physician

The pivotal figure in medicine in the United States throughout the twentieth century has been the physician. The history of the physician supply in the United States has been variable, reflecting periods of undersupply and oversupply. The early part of the century was characterized by a relatively high physicians-to-population ratio of over 170 physicians for every 100,000 people in the United States. Significant changes in educational and licensing requirements beginning in 1912 forced the closure of many medical diploma mills, decreased the number of practicing physicians, and severely restricted the production of physicians, with a subsequent decline in the ratio to about 130:100,000 in 1940. More recently, as the supply of physicians has increased, there has again been concern about a "glut" of physicians. As is the case with uncertainty about the appropriate number of hospital beds, part of the problem may lie in a continuing inability to determine and agree on either a proper physicians-to-population ratio or a distribution of physicians that would be conducive to some equally elusive optimal level of medical care.

Dental Care

For the majority of people in the United States in 1900, dental care was virtually nonexistent. There were only 25,000 dentists in the entire country, or 33 for every 100,000 people. While the number of dentists and the dentists-to-population ratio increased and remained steady for a number of years, in the past 20 years the ratio has actually decreased, perhaps reflecting a decreased demand for dental care as a result of flouridation of most major public water supplies. Today there are approximately 130,000 dentists, creating a ratio of about 46:100,000.

Conclusion

Even this introductory overview of selected population, health, and medical care characteristics of the United States reflects dramatic changes in the life and death experience of the nation. The events and changes described here have not been uniformly experienced across the nation; cumulative or aggregate national experience with health, death, and medical care at any particular moment is composed of a mosaic of geographic variations. Death rates, major threats to health, the major causes of death, and the provision of medical care have not been and today are not uniformly distributed from place to place. In this volume we examine the historical and geographic variation in national mortality and medical care experience during the twentieth century and assess the most recent patterns as the twenty-first century approaches.

This review has several foci. In order to provide a context for examining morbidity, mortality, and health care, we begin by discussing general trends and geographic variations in selected population characteristics, including age structure, racial mixture, population density, and per capita income. Attention is then directed to geographic and temporal patterns of the mortality experience in the United States. Our assessment of mortality patterns is necessarily limited in terms of both number and scale. It has been necessary to select a relatively few causes of death and the associated mortality rates. The selection was based primarily upon the relative significance of each cause at some time during the twentieth century. Among the items included for discussion and description are general characteristics of infant mortality and specific patterns of death related to tuberculosis, heart and cerebrovascular diseases, selected cancers, and motor vehicle accidents. In addition, we treat the major epidemics of influenza and AIDS.

Subsequently, we examine changes in selected components of the medical care sector. The changing production, supply, and distribution of physicians and dentists, as well as changes in the supply and distribu-

tion of general and mental hospital beds, are displayed and discussed.

Information on population, mortality, and medical care is presented and illustrated on a state-by-state basis. Certainly, choosing state-based data masks important differences which occur within each state, and it might be argued that a more detailed analysis would provide more insight. The purpose of this book, however, is to illustrate the state and regional experience of the United States. Also important to the decision was the availability of data. We made our decision to assess patterns at the interstate level on the basis of the availability of data over a considerable period of time. Even at this level, uniformly collected vital statistics did not become available for each and every state until completion of the Death Registration Area in 1933. We hope that the geographic and historic perspectives adopted here will contribute to an understanding of important dimensions of twentieth-century life and death in the United States.

2

General Population Characteristics

Population Growth in the Twentieth Century

As mentioned in Chapter 1, an estimated 270 million people are expected to live in the United States by the year 2000. In 1990 the population of the United States was approximately 250 million, more than 3 times larger than the population of 76 million people that was recorded in the 1900 Census (Figure 2.1). In turn, the 1990 population was more than 15 times larger than the 5 million population of a century earlier. Though population growth has been sustained during the twentieth century, it has slowed considerably as compared to growth in the preceding century, and it has also fluctuated considerably.

In the early part of the century, from 1900 through 1915, the population grew by about 8 percent every 5 years, that is, by between 6 and 7 million people. From 1916 through 1920, the combined effects of World War I, which accounted for over 100,000 battle and battle-related deaths among United States personnel, and, more important, the influenza epidemic of 1918–1919, which resulted in a little more than 500,000 deaths in the United States, contributed to a decrease in the population growth rate to only 4 percent (Figure 2.2). While there was some recovery in the 1920s, population increases of about 3 to 4 million people, or only 3 percent, occurred in the 1930s, the

period of the most severe economic depression of the twentieth century.

The period of World War II, 1941–1945, is especially notable because there was actually a population decrease of 0.5 percent, or 640,000 people. This circumstance was caused in part by two factors: a decreased birth rate resulting from the deployment of millions of young men and women and, more important, over 400,000 deaths related to the war. Several immediate post-World War II periods were marked by rather substantial population increases of between 10 and 12 million people, or about 7 percent during each 5-year increment.

Since 1965 the percentage increases in total population measured over 5-year intervals have declined substantially once again, averaging 4 percent and reflecting increases of between 8 and 9 million people. However, in the interval from 1986 to 1990, the increase was less than 4 percent. It would appear that the United States will continue to experience a modest population growth rate through the end of the twentieth century.

Population Pyramids

The demographic structure of the U.S. population during this century can also be examined in the context of the age/gender population pyramids depicted in Figures 2.3 to 2.6. In the year 1900, the population struc-

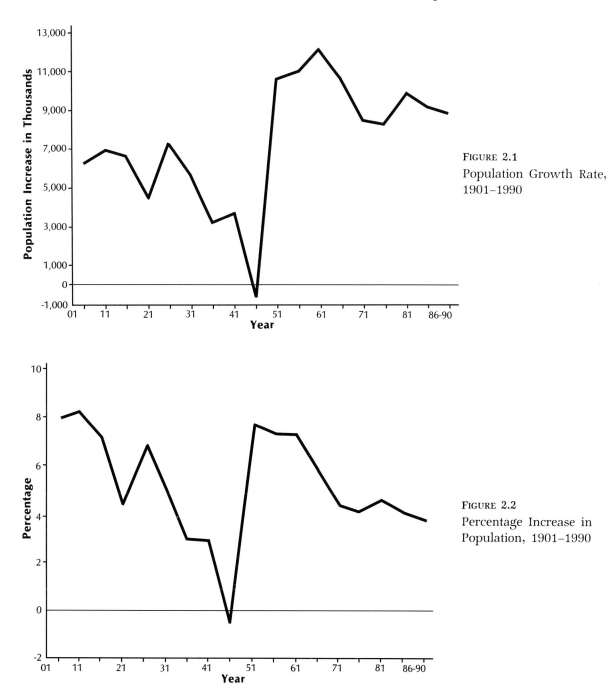

FIGURE 2.1
Population Growth Rate,
1901–1990

FIGURE 2.2
Percentage Increase in
Population, 1901–1990

ture of the country was similar to that of many developing nations of today (Figure 2.3). The younger age cohorts (less than 5 years old, aged 5 to 9, and aged 10 to 14) were the most numerous for both females and males. In addition, the population under age 30 was substantially higher than at any other time during this century. There was also a very limited population over 65 years old.

By 1930, both the effects of World War I and the beginnings of the Great Depression were reflected in the U.S. population age pyramid (Figure 2.4). The less-than-5-years-old age cohorts for both females and

males had decreased substantially in comparison to most other youthful cohorts. There were also fewer males than would have otherwise been expected, in the age cohorts that had participated in World War I. As also examined in Chapter 4 in the discussion of influenza, many Americans between the ages of 20 and 40 died during the winter of 1918–19. This effect is reflected in the 1930 age pyramid.

Historical and economic events and trends continued to assist in forming the structure of the U.S. population. By 1960, the effects of two world wars, the Great Depression, and the post-World War II baby boom were

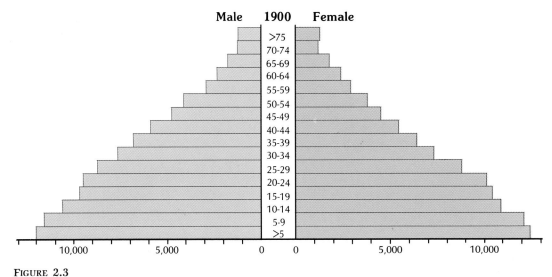

FIGURE 2.3
Population Pyramid, 1900

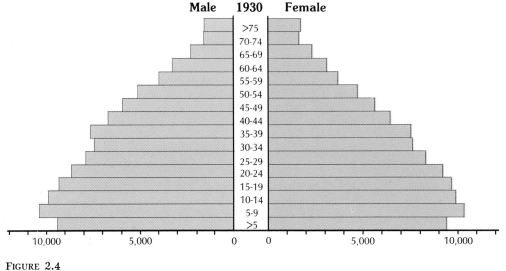

FIGURE 2.4
Population Pyramid, 1930

clearly visible in the context of a population pyramid (Figure 2.5). The large indentation in the 20-to-40 U.S. age cohorts in 1960 was a result of lower birth rates during the Depression as well as losses and lower birth rates during World War II. The dramatic population increases for two decades after World War II are clearly shown in the 1960 population pyramid. By 1960, the three largest age cohorts for females and males represented many persons less than 15 years old. It should also be noted from examination of the 1960 pyramid that persons in the several age cohorts more than 65 years old were more numerous than before. Better medical services and the advent of modern antibiotics had contributed to longer life spans.

The 1988 population age pyramid was also quite different from the earlier periods shown (Figure 2.6). The "baby boomer" age cohorts continued to be the most numerous age groups within the United States. Birth

rates declined during the Vietnam era and the economically difficult times of the 1970s. Many of the "boomer" group had also opted to have children later in life than had their parents. Two other trends of importance with respect to population structure show up in the 1988 pyramid. First, the 1988 U.S. population over 50 years old was larger than ever before, both in terms of absolute numbers and as a percentage of the total. Again, because of continued progress in modern health care delivery, people were simply living longer. The second aspect of the age structure related to the over-50 group is that there were proportionately more females than males for all the cohorts over 50 years of age by the end of the 1980s.

In general, the population pyramid of the United States in 1988 resembled that of a developed European country more than ever before. Clearly, the country had passed through an epidemiological transition.

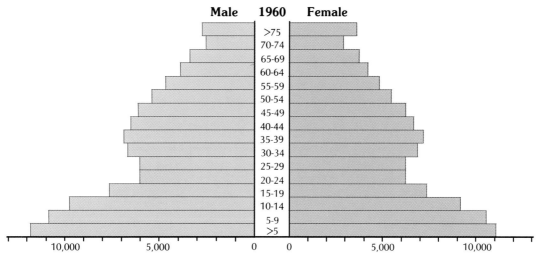

FIGURE 2.5
Population Pyramid, 1960

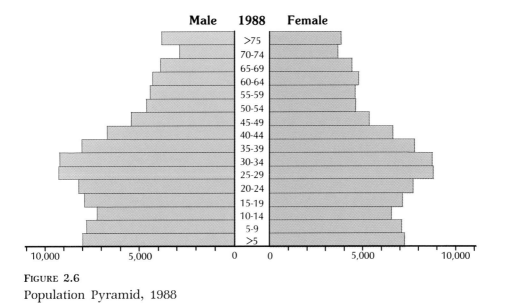

FIGURE 2.6
Population Pyramid, 1988

Population Density

The relative geographic stability of the United States in terms of total land area coupled with the increase of population has contributed to a steady increase in the population density of the United States, as measured in terms of number of persons per square mile. Overall, the nation's population density has more than tripled since 1900, when it was about 22 persons per square mile. The current geographic and demographic characteristics of the United States as a whole translate into a population density of about 70 persons per square mile. However, based on the geographic configuration of 1900—that is, excluding the areas and populations of states added since 1900, namely, Arizona, Alaska, and Hawaii—today there are over 86 persons per square mile, almost quadruple the density of the same area in 1900.

The population is not evenly distributed across the country, and certain states are more densely populated than others. Even within a state, the population may be concentrated in relatively small areas composed of large cities and larger metropolitan areas. Thus, much of the increase in density is related to the population growth of the largest cities in each state. Nevertheless, the individual population density of each state when compared with figures for other states does provide an indication of the relative distribution of the population across the country.

1900. In 1900 a number of states had fewer than 2 persons per square mile, including Idaho, Montana, and Wyoming in the Northwest and Nevada and New Mexico in the Southwest (Figure 2.7). Nevada, which had only 42,000 people in 1900, is particularly notable; it had fewer than 0.5 person per square mile. Utah,

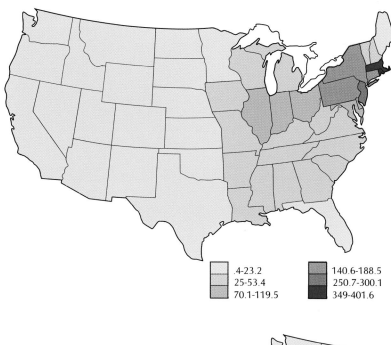

FIGURE 2.7

Population Density (Persons per square mile), 1900

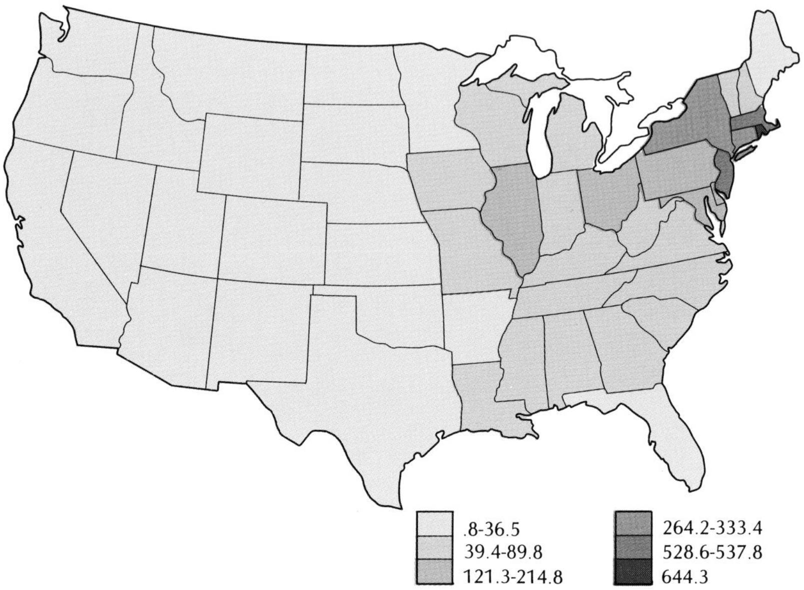

.4-23.2	140.6-188.5
25-53.4	250.7-300.1
70.1-119.5	349-401.6

FIGURE 2.8

Population Density (Persons per square mile), 1930

.8-36.5	264.2-333.4
39.4-89.8	528.6-537.8
121.3-214.8	644.3

North Dakota, and South Dakota had 5 or fewer persons per square mile.

The most densely settled states were those in the Northeast. Rhode Island was the smallest in terms of area but it had 425,000 people in 1900 and more than 400 persons per square mile. Another small state, Massachusetts, averaged about 350 persons per square mile, and New Jersey had over 250 persons per square mile. Other states in the region, including Connecticut and New York, had densities of over 150 people per square mile, again with most people located in the largest cities. Nearby, more rural states, such as New Hampshire, Vermont, and Maine, had between 20 and 50 persons per square mile.

1930. While population densities increased along with the increasing population of the country, the general characteristics of the 1930 pattern (Figure 2.8) were virtually the same as those in 1900. Again, the lowest population densities were found in the Northwest and the Southwest. Nevada more than doubled its population to 92,000 between 1900 and 1930, yet still had fewer than 1 person per square mile. Arizona, New Mexico, and Montana had fewer than 4 persons per square mile. Again, the northeastern states—including Rhode Island with a density of almost 650 persons per square mile, New Jersey with 538 persons per square mile, and Massachusetts with 529 persons per square mile—were the most densely populated. In the far

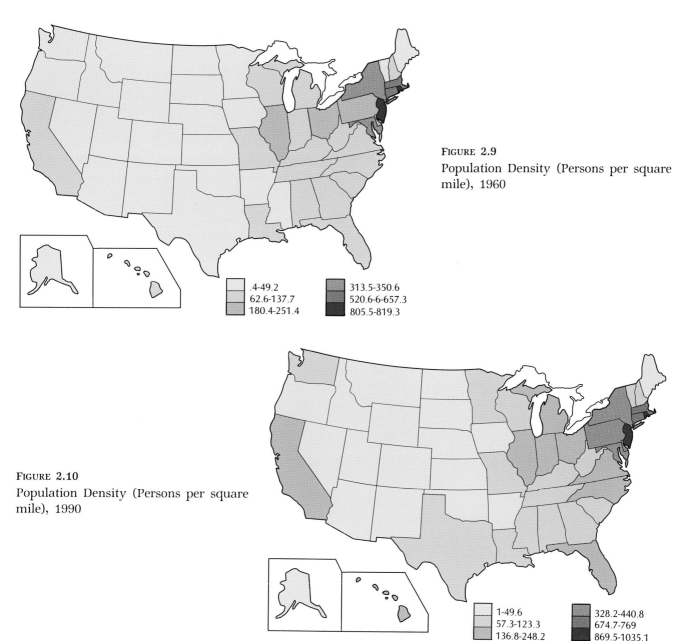

FIGURE 2.9
Population Density (Persons per square mile), 1960

.4-49.2	313.5-350.6
62.6-137.7	520.6-6-657.3
180.4-251.4	805.5-819.3

FIGURE 2.10
Population Density (Persons per square mile), 1990

1-49.6	328.2-440.8
57.3-123.3	674.7-769
136.8-248.2	869.5-1035.1

West, California's population density increased almost fourfold between 1900 and 1930, from almost 10 to 37 persons per square mile. Washington also experienced a threefold increase in population density, from 8 persons per square mile in 1900 to about 24 in 1930. Oklahoma matched this increase, moving from 11 persons per square mile in 1900 to 35 in 1930. Florida was close behind, increasing in population density from about 10 persons per square mile to 27 during the 30-year period. Even the more densely settled states, such as New York and especially New Jersey, experienced considerable increases in population density. New York's population density almost doubled, from 153 to 264 persons per square mile. New Jersey more than

doubled in population density, from 251 to 538 persons per square mile. Minimal increases in population density (that is, less than 15 percent), occurred in states such as Iowa, Maine, and Vermont.

1960. In 1960 Rhode Island, with almost 900,000 residents and 819 persons per square mile, and New Jersey, with over 6 million people and a population density of 806, were the most densely settled states (Figure 2.9). Also in the highest-density quartile were Massachusetts with 657 persons per square mile and Connecticut with 521. The new state of Alaska, with over 0.5 million square miles of land area and a population density of fewer than 0.5 person per square

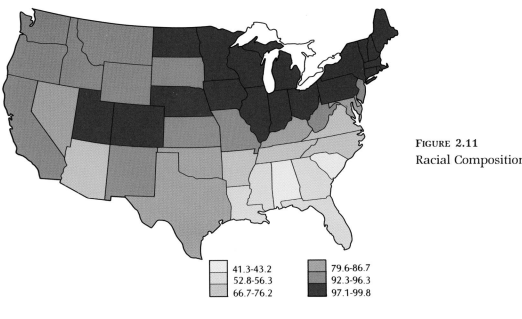

FIGURE 2.11
Racial Composition (Percent White), 1900

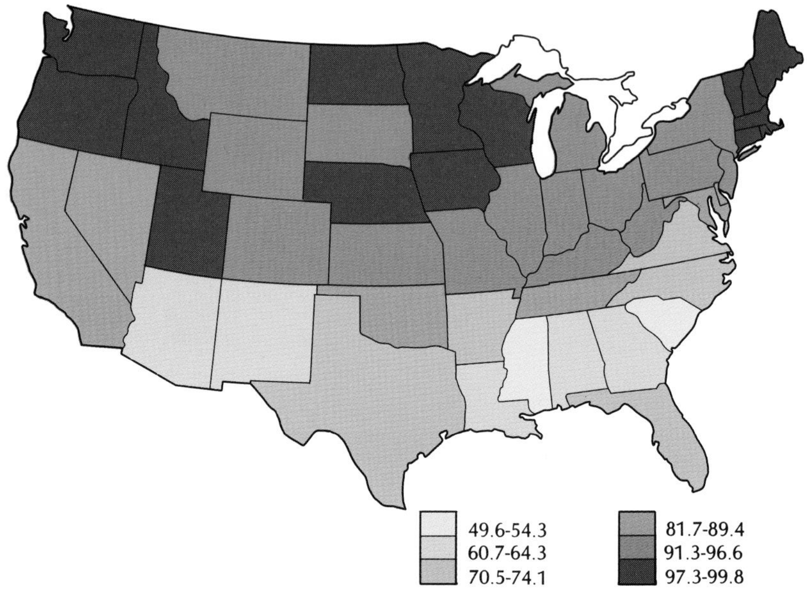

41.3-43.2	79.6-86.7
52.8-56.3	92.3-96.3
66.7-76.2	97.1-99.8

FIGURE 2.12
Racial Composition (Percent White), 1930

49.6-54.3	81.7-89.4
60.7-64.3	91.3-96.6
70.5-74.1	97.3-99.8

mile, was the least densely settled area of the country. Nevada had fewer than 3 persons per square mile in 1960. In the industrial heartland of the country, the highly urbanized states of Ohio, with 237 persons per square mile, and Illinois, with 180, were the most densely populated. The population densities of the Dakotas remained low, about 9 persons per square mile, virtually unchanged from 1930 to 1960. On the other hand, the population density of Florida more than tripled. It increased from 27 to 92 persons per square mile. Arizona's population density increased from 4 to 12 persons per square mile. The population density of California almost tripled, increasing from 37 to over 100 persons per square mile.

1990. In 1990 the geographic pattern of state population densities still showed some major features which have been consistent since 1900 (Figure 2.10). The most densely populated states were still the ones in the Northeast. New Jersey is now the most densely settled state and was the first to reach a population density of over 1,000 persons per square mile. Rhode Island's population density remained high, at about 870 persons per square mile, but failed to keep pace with the increase in New Jersey since 1960. Massachusetts, Connecticut, Maryland, and New York were also among the most densely populated states. North Dakota and South Dakota had 1990 population densities of about 9 persons per square mile, still virtually unchanged from 1930.

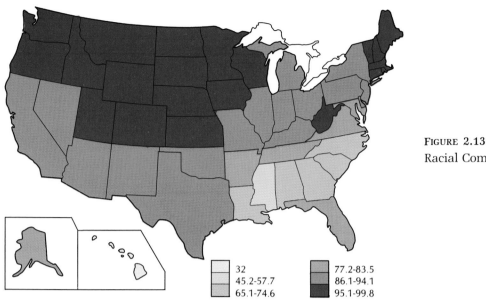

FIGURE 2.13
Racial Composition (Percent White), 1960

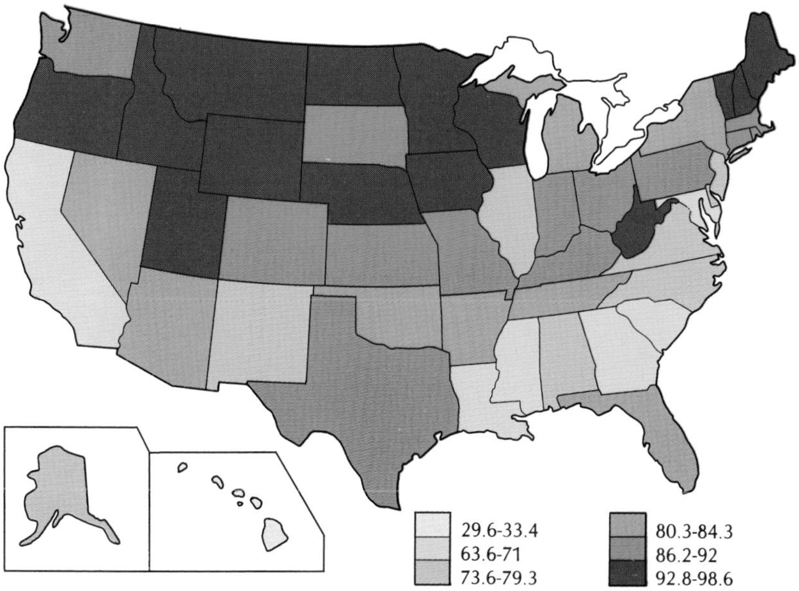

32	77.2-83.5
45.2-57.7	86.1-94.1
65.1-74.6	95.1-99.8

FIGURE 2.14
Racial Composition (Percent White), 1990

29.6-33.4	80.3-84.3
63.6-71	86.2-92
73.6-79.3	92.8-98.6

Nevada's population density had increased by 250 percent since 1960 but was still only 9 persons per square mile. Arizona increased in population density to 32 persons per square mile, an increase of about 180 percent over the 1960 figure. California, the most populous state with over 29 million people, experienced a 90 percent increase in population density between 1960 and 1990, increasing to more than 190 persons per square mile. Though the population density of Alaska increased by 150 percent between 1960 and 1990, it remained the lowest of any state, at 1 person per square mile.

Toward the Twenty-First Century. Unless some unforeseen and major changes take place in the expected population increase and distribution in the next few years, the population density pattern in the year 2000 should be quite similar to that of 1990. States that have experienced considerable recent population growth are Nevada, which increased 50 percent between 1980 and 1990; Arizona, with a 35 percent increase; Florida, with 33 percent; and California, with 26 percent. These states can be expected to reflect the greatest increases in population density. At the same time, if recent population trends continue over the next decade, states such as West Virginia (which lost 8 percent of its population between 1980 and 1990), Iowa (which has 5 percent fewer people), and Illinois (which has 3 percent fewer) can be expected to decline in population density.

Racial Composition

Just as the population densities of states vary considerably, so too do their racial compositions. Moreover, when measured in terms of the proportions of blacks, whites, and other races, though general national geographical patterns remain similar, the racial compositions of many individual states have changed considerably over the past 90 years. It should be noted that before 1930 persons of the "Mexican race" were included in the "white" classification. Therefore, the percentage of whites is overestimated in the earlier national and state totals. Bearing this in mind, the proportions of black, white, and other population groups have remained relatively stable throughout the twentieth century.

In 1900 approximately 88 percent of the total population was classified as "white" (including the "Mexican race"), compared to 84 percent in 1990 (Figure 2.11). While there was a decline in the first half of the century due to the surge of immigrants from European countries, today the black population as a percentage of the total is about 12 percent, the same as it was in 1900. Particularly notable is the recent surge in the number of Asians living in the United States. Though Asians still make up just under 3 percent of the total population, it is estimated that their number increased by more than 90 percent in the 1980s, from a total of under 4 million to almost 7 million people. Among the key factors contributing to this increase was a 1965 change in the immigration law, removing restrictions on Asians which had been in place since early in the century. As a result, the number of Asian-Americans jumped from 0.9 million in 1960 to 1.4 million in 1970, to 3.8 million in 1980, and to 7.3 million in 1990.

As illustrated in Figures 2.11 to 2.14, there are substantial differences from state to state in terms of the racial characteristics of the populations. Moreover, dramatic changes in the geographic patterns of racial composition of the United States have taken place during the twentieth century.

1900. Reflecting the legacy of large slave populations, in 1900 blacks were still residing predominantly in the southeastern United States, below the Mason-Dixon Line (Figure 2.11). Although whites were in the majority in many of these states, such as Alabama, Florida, Louisiana, and Georgia, the total populations composed almost equal proportions of blacks and whites. Particularly notable were Mississippi (with 59 percent blacks) and South Carolina (57 percent), in which the black populations were in the clear majority in 1900. In other states, such as Arkansas and North Carolina, blacks constituted about one-third of the total populations. By contrast, in most states to the north and west

of the southeastern region the populations were virtually all white. For example, over 98 percent of the populations of states such as Connecticut, Illinois, Massachusetts, Michigan, and New York were white. In fact, 28 of the 47 states in 1900 had populations which were at least 95 percent white. Notable concentrations of Native Americans were found in the Arizona territory (23 percent) and in the state of Nevada (16 percent).

1930. By 1930, some substantial changes had taken place, marked by declines in percentages of blacks in most southern states as they migrated northward to find jobs in the industrial Northeast (Figure 2.12). Still, with the exception of Texas and Maryland, most states outside the Deep South had relatively small percentages of black populations. By this time, blacks were a majority only in Mississippi, and this was by a fractional percentage (50.2 percent). The percentages of blacks as proportions of the total population decreased more than 10 percent between 1900 and 1930 in Alabama, Florida, Georgia, Louisiana, and South Carolina. Though blacks still constituted less than 5 percent of the total populations, their percentages increased in states such as Illinois, Michigan, Ohio, and Pennsylvania. This trend reflected the migration from the southern states, a movement pattern which was to continue for the next 30 years.

1960. By 1960, due in large part to migration of blacks from the state and to an influx of whites from the North, the percentage of the total Florida population that was white increased to over 80 percent (Figure 2.13). In 1900 the white population had been only 56 percent of the total. The percentages of blacks in the populations of most southern states continued to decline between 1930 and 1960. By 1960, there were no states in which the black populations constituted a majority. The largest percentages of blacks remained in Mississippi (42 percent) and South Carolina (46 percent). In the large industrial states to the north—such as Illinois (10.3 percent), Michigan (9.2 percent), New York (8.5 percent), Ohio (8.1 percent) and Pennsylvania (7.5 percent)—the black populations increased to sizable minorities. Between 1930 and 1960 in California the percentage of blacks increased fourfold, from 1.4 percent to 5.6 percent of the total population. Populations of states in the far West (such as Washington and Oregon), in the midwest (such as Kansas, Nebraska, and Colorado), and in New England remained over 95 percent white.

1990. Overall, the 1990 geographic pattern of racial composition in the United States has remained similar to the pattern observed in 1960, although sizable increases in the percentages of blacks as proportions of total state populations have occurred in states such as

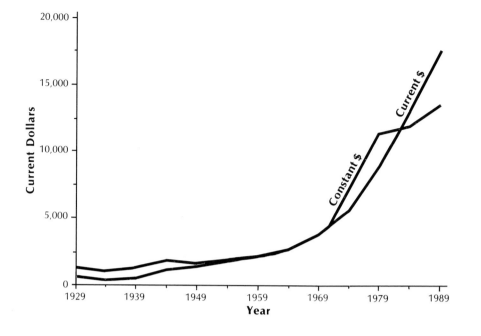

FIGURE 2.15
Per Capita Personal Income,
1929–1989

Maryland (with an increase from 17 to 26 percent) and New York (from 8 to 16 percent). (See Figure 2.14.) Most changes were more moderate, as in Illinois (from 10 to 16 percent), Michigan (from 9 to 15 percent), and Ohio (from 8 to 11 percent). Similarly, the percentage decreases in black populations as proportions of total populations in southern states were moderate. In Alabama, for example, in 1990 the black population constituted almost 27 percent of the total population, as compared to 30 percent in 1960. In Mississippi the percentage decreased from 42 to 36 percent, and in South Carolina it decreased from 35 to 30 percent. Particularly notable is California, the most populous state (with almost 30 million people), in which Asians constituted 9.6 percent of the population in 1990, surpassing the black population of 7.4 percent.

Toward the Twenty-First Century. Substantial changes in the racial composition of individual states continue to take place, yet remnants of the geographic pattern of racial composition of the United States observed in 1900 are apparent, a legacy inherited from over 125 years ago. The proportions of blacks in the populations of most northern and western states have increased, but the states in the southeastern part of the country continue to have the largest proportions of blacks. There is also some indication of a reverse migration of blacks, moving from northern states to the South, paralleling the recent general pattern of white migration. Though recent immigration of Asians has altered the racial composition of many states, the total impact on the population structure has been minimal, with the exception of California.

The shift toward racial and ethnic minorities since 1980 is believed to be the sharpest which has occurred in the twentieth century. Today, almost one of every four Americans is identified with an African, native American, Asian, or Hispanic ancestry. In 1980, one in five Americans had such a minority background. Some observers of the long-term and recent trends mentioned above have suggested that what is happening is "the dawning of the first universal nation." At the same time, however, there are predictions of increasing polarization and turmoil among an increasingly diverse racial and ethnic population.

Per Capita Income

Information on per capita personal income was first collected and calculated in 1929. Except during the Great Depression, on average the personal income of each individual has increased (Figure 2.15). However, the increase in personal income is not so great when a standard measure is used which incorporates the decline in purchasing power of the dollar. Though per capita personal income has increased rather precipitously since 1969, the value of the dollar is considerably less due to rising costs. In 1989, the average per capita personal income in the United States was about $17,600, yet in terms of 1982 dollar purchasing power, per capita income was only $13,500. The discrepancy would be even greater if the earlier standard of the 1958 dollar were used. Thus, while per capita income in terms of current dollars continues to escalate, purchasing power has stagnated.

Though living costs and purchasing power of a dollar vary widely, the per capita personal income figures do provide an indication of the regional variation in the wealth of individuals within the nation.

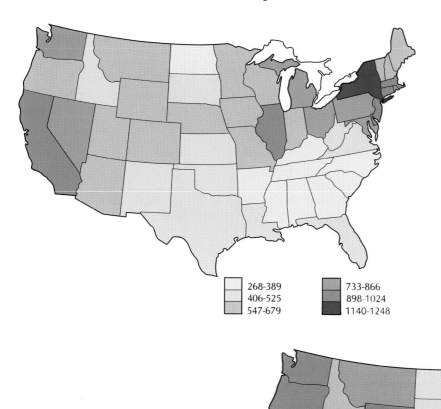

FIGURE 2.16
Per Capita Personal Income, 1929

268-389	733-866
406-525	898-1024
547-679	1140-1248

FIGURE 2.17

Per Capita Personal Income, 1949

710-967	1394-1505
1021-1219	1584-1778
1247-1373	2062

1929. In 1929, annual per capita personal income by state ranged from $268 to $1,248, certainly modest by present-day figures (Figure 2.16). However, it must be remembered that well-built houses could be purchased for less than $4,000 and automobiles for less than $1,000. In any event, there was considerable regional variation in the geographic distribution of per capita personal incomes. Particularly notable is the group of southeastern states. Of the nine states in the lowest annual per capita income category in 1929 ($268 to $389), eight were in the Southeast. South Carolina had the lowest per capita income, $268, and Mississippi had $282. This core group of low-income states was bounded by states in the next lowest income group, in

which annual per capita income ranged from $406 to $525 per year. Included in this group were Texas, Louisiana, Florida, Virginia, and West Virginia. New York state had the highest per capita income, $1,140 per year. The remainder of the manufacturing states—Illinois, Michigan, Ohio, and Pennsylvania—had average per capita incomes ranging from $733 to $1,024. Of the states in the far West, California residents had the highest per capita income, $973.

1949. By 1949, average per capita income had increased to about $1,380 (Figure 2.17). As in 1900, Mississippi again had the lowest average ($710), just over one-half the national average, followed by Alabama

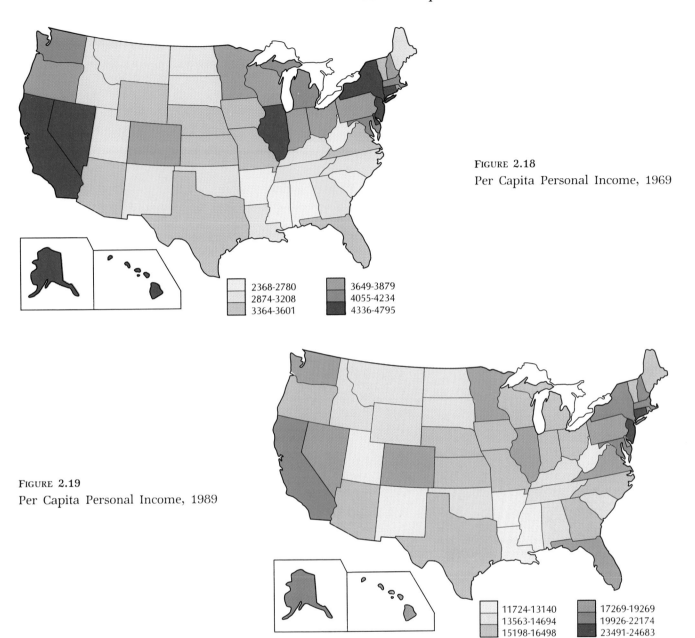

FIGURE 2.18
Per Capita Personal Income, 1969

2368-2780	3649-3879
2874-3208	4055-4234
3364-3601	4336-4795

FIGURE 2.19
Per Capita Personal Income, 1989

11724-13140	17269-19269
13563-14694	19926-22174
15198-16498	23491-24683

with $835. The average per capita incomes of North Carolina and South Carolina were also under $900 in 1949. The states with the highest per capita incomes were widely distributed, from Delaware ($1,770) and New York ($1,706) to California ($1,720) and Nevada ($1,778).

1969. Average per capita income in the United States had increased to just over $3,800 by 1969 (Figure 2.18). As in 1900 and 1930, Mississippi, with a per capita income of about $2,370, ranked lowest. Arkansas, with a per capita income of $2,600, replaced Alabama ($2,725) as the second lowest. West Virginia ($2,764) and South Carolina ($2,780) remained in the lowest

quartile of states in terms of per capita income. Outside the Southeast, New Mexico had an average per capita income of $2,888, South Dakota had $2,948, and North Dakota had $2,993.

At the other end of the per capita income spectrum were states such as Connecticut, with the highest average of all ($4,795), closely followed by Alaska ($4,642) and New York ($4,574). Illinois ($4,336) and Michigan ($4055) in the Midwest; Nevada ($4,475) in the Southwest; and California ($4,485), and Hawaii ($4,411) in the far West also had high average per capita incomes.

1989. Between 1969 and 1989, the average per capita income in the United States increased from about

1989. Between 1969 and 1989, the average per capita income in the United States increased from about $3,800 to $17,600, some 450 percent (Figure 2.19). Connecticut ($24,683), New Jersey ($23,778), Massachusetts ($22,174), Alaska ($21,656), and New York ($21,073) had per capita incomes which were at least $3,400 higher than the national average. Consistent with previous years considered here, Mississippi ($11,724) again had the lowest per capita income, almost $6,000 less than the national average. West Virginia ($12,345), Louisiana ($12,921), and Arkansas ($12,901) had per capita incomes at least $5,000 less than the national average. Outside the Southeast, North Dakota, South Dakota, Idaho, New Mexico, and Utah also had very low per capita incomes.

Keeping in mind regional differences in living costs and the associated differences in buying power of the dollar, a consistent pattern of relative poverty can be seen throughout the twentieth century, dominated by a concentration of low per capita incomes throughout much of the southeastern United States and in "outlier" states such as North Dakota and South Dakota. All these statistical trends—population growth; population density, racial composition, and per capita income—have affected health and disease patterns in the United States.

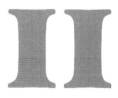

Geographic Patterns
of Infirmity
and Mortality

3

Lingering Morbidity Problems: Tuberculosis and Influenza

TUBERCULOSIS

We begin our examination of disease mortality with one of the most historically significant diseases: tuberculosis (TB). According to World Health Organization estimates, there are approximately 20 million people with active cases of TB in the world today, and an additional 50 million to 100 million people, primarily children, are infected annually. Worldwide mortality due to TB is between 3 million and 5 million persons annually. Tuberculosis continues to be a major medical problem in most developing countries. In contrast, in the mid-twentieth century in the United States, researchers suggested that TB would become a medical curiosity by the beginning of the twenty-first century. Unfortunately, it has now become apparent that this will not be the case. There are very disturbing findings of TB resurgence among certain population groups in the United States. In addition, the strains of TB that are now appearing seem to be resistant to much current drug treatment.

History

TB appears to be as old as humanity itself. It appears in skeletal remains of prehistoric humans found in Germany dating back to 8000 B.C. and in Egyptian skeletons dating from 2500 to 1000 B.C. Ancient Hindu and Chinese writings also document the presence of TB. Evidence for the antiquity of the disease in the Americas comes from an Inca mummy of an 8-year-old boy from southern Peru who lived about A.D. 700. The child had evidence of long-standing bone and soft tissue TB.

Historically, TB has been known by a number of names. The Greek physician Hippocrates (470–377 B.C.), known as the father of medicine, named it "phthisis" (thi-sis) meaning "to waste away," which reflected the wasting of the body caused by respiratory TB. In the eighteenth and nineteenth centuries the disease was commonly called "consumption" or "consumption of the lung." The term "tuberculosis" derives from observations by a German physician and anatomist, Franciscus Sylvius (1614–1672), who, in the latter part of the seventeenth century divulged finding in phthisis victims' lungs, small rounded masses or nodules which he named "tubercles." Other terms applied to TB include "scrofula," "asthenia," "tabes," "bronchitis," "inflammation of the lungs," "hectic fever," "gastric fever," and "lupus." The term "white plague" derived from the pasty-white pallor of TB victims and was coined at a time when TB was believed to threaten the very survival of Europeans.

Perhaps the most captivating description of TB was written by John Bunyan (1628–1688), author of *Pilgrim's Progress*. In *The Life and Death of Mr. Badman*, Bunyan wrote "THE CAPTAIN OF ALL THESE MEN OF DEATH that came against him to take him away, was the Consumption, for it was that that brought him down to the grave."

Throughout history, TB has been no respector of persons. Among those who succumbed to it were such personages as Louis XIII, king of France (reigned 1610–1643). The English poet John Keats (1795–1821), who died of TB at the age of 26, wrote in 1819: "Youth grows pale, and spectre thin, and dies." The long-suffering Italian violinist, Nicolo Paganini (1782–1840), played from his deathbed before dying of TB (and syphilis). The Polish composer and pianist Frederic Chopin (1810–1849) unsuccessfully sought a cure for his TB in Majorca. Consumption was particularly harsh to the literary Bronte family of England. Charlotte (1816–1855) was most famous for *Jane Eyre*, Emily (1818–1848) wrote *Wuthering Heights*, and Anne (1820–1849) was the author of *Agnes Grey* and *Tenant of Wildfell Hall*. All died of consumption. In the United States, Henry David Thoreau (1817–1862), who was most famous for the experiment that led to publication of his *Walden*, died of consumption in Concord, Massachusetts, shortly after returning from a futile search for a cure in Minnesota, a popular place for the treatment of consumptives. Nathaniel Hawthorne (1804–1864), author of *Twice-Told Tales* and *The Scarlett Letter*, lived for years with TB, yet it killed him in the end. Other notable Americans who died of consumption were John Harvard (1607–1638), the clergyman and scholar for whom Harvard College was named; the explorer Jacques Marquette (1637–1675); Stephen Crane (1871–1900), author of *The Red Badge of Courage*; Paul Lawrence Dunbar (1872–1906), a poet who was the son of an escaped slave and the author of *Slow through the Dark*; and Christopher Mathewson (1880–1925), one of the most renowned baseball players of the early twentieth century.

Etiology

The "classic" TB is a predominately chronic, communicable disease caused by the pathogen *Mycobacterium tuberculosis*. In the vast majority of cases the lungs are involved, but any organ or tissue in the human body may be affected. Wherever the bacilli invade the human tissue, they evoke a characteristic reaction from the body in the form of a granule (granuloma) known as a "tubercle."

The Tubercle Bacillus

The tubercle bacillus is a microscopic rod-shaped bacterium which grows slowly and may remain dormant in humans after a growth period of several weeks. The dormant period may extend for months, years, or even the lifetime of the infected individual. Therefore, despite being infected with the TB bacillus, the individual may live for an extended period or even a lifetime in apparent good health.

The TB bacilli grow optimally in parts of the body that have the highest oxygen supplies, such as the lungs. Historically, approximately 92 to 94 percent of all clinically recognized TB is pulmonary. However, bacilli "seeded" throughout the body tend to multiply at the sites of greatest oxygen tension, namely, the apices or tips of the lungs and kidneys and well-vascularized areas like the growing ends of long bones. In this manner, TB may develop in bones and other tissues without the pulmonary form of the disease. However, the primary tubercular lesion is most likely to occur in the lower or middle portions of the lung because these areas have a much greater volume than the apices and are therefore more likely to be the sites where airborne tubercle bacilli lodge.

Modes of Transmission

The bacillus is most commonly transmitted from an infected person to others by way of infected droplets. Droplet nuclei are developed and discharged when the diseased person coughs, sneezes, speaks, or even sings. Moreover, the tubercle bacilli are so durable and resistant to drying that they may remain viable for months in dust and on articles of daily use. The very small droplet nuclei (in the range of 1 to 10 microns) may remain suspended in the air for hours. Only droplet nuclei less than 10 microns in diameter are small enough to reach the alveoli of the lungs. Thus, the most common entry to the body is through the airways of the nose and mouth.

Other methods of transmission are possible, but their potential for infection is small. For example, ingestion of the *Mycobacterium bovis*, a tubercle bacillus found in cow milk, was once common. In the United States this source of infection was eliminated by a 1917 federal program of the Bureau of Animal Industry. Dairy herds were carefully tested through examination of milk supplies, and tuberculosis cows were eliminated. However, even when it was more common in the United States, this type of transmission was much less frequent than was airborne person-to-person spread.

It is difficult, though possible, for tubercle bacilli to reach the alveoli of the lung from a contaminated object. Of course, a person may ingest the tubercle bacilli by making oral contact with contaminated hands or by introducing a contaminated object into the mouth. However, most bacilli will be eliminated by saliva and the number of tubercle bacilli acquired in this manner would be too few to produce progressive TB by way of the intestinal tract. Nevertheless, all food handlers, such as restaurant and cafeteria workers, are tested annually for tuberculosis.

Epidemiology

The epidemiology of TB is a complex and still incompletely unraveled mystery. The times necessary to achieve a low degree of TB incidence and mortality are believed to be inversely proportional to the *degree of urbanization*. This is because factors which increase the opportunity of infection include large-scale human migration, crowds, and economic hardship (which cause cramped living quarters, insufficient food intake, and unsanitary living conditions). These factors, though common in urban areas, are also frequently found in certain segments of the population living in rural areas. The TB epidemic can be expected to be more severe and to run its course more rapidly in urban than in surrounding rural areas. However, as the rural and urban areas become more integrated through improved transportation and increased suburbanization, epidemics can be expected to encompass both rural and urban areas.

Endemic Tuberculosis

The presence of TB in pre-Columbian North America is a matter of some debate. For example, researchers early in the twentieth century concluded that tuberculosis was uncommon. Very few North American prehistoric skeletal remains with indications of TB had been unearthed and adequately assessed at the turn of the century. The endemic TB among Native Americans on reservations was attributed to a greater degree of susceptibility due to lack of contact with the disease rather than to the conditions prevailing on the reservations.

By the mid-twentieth century, accumulation of additional information and increased knowledge about TB led to the conclusion that there may have been more pre-Columbian tuberculosis than previously thought. Today, it is generally agreed that TB did exist at relatively low levels among prehistoric populations, including Native Americans. However, important questions—"Where?" "Why?" "How?"—remain largely unanswered, and inferences about the geographic distribution of TB and related environmental factors are far from secure for this early time period.

The first North American peak of TB probably occurred about the year 1800 in the metropolitan areas of the Atlantic seaboard. The TB mortality rate must have been over 1,000 and probably reached 1,500 per 100,000 population. The peak mortality rate in New England is estimated to have been 1,600 per year in 1800. Between 1810 and 1820, Boston recorded a rate of 489 per 100,000 population. Other cities had similarly high rates: New York City (1804–1808), 580 per 100,000; Philadelphia (1811–1820), 501 per 100,000; and Charleston, South Carolina (1822–1830), 400 per 100,000. In most areas, TB accounted for between 20 and 25 percent of all deaths.

Though TB was the leading cause of death throughout the nineteenth century and the beginning of the twentieth, it was apparently already on the decrease as early as 1840. By 1896, the death rate from TB was 241 per 100,000 population in New York City and 237 per 100,000 in Philadelphia. Within a span of less than a century, the mortality rate had been more than halved, without the benefit of public health or medical measures and in a period of increasing urbanization. The point to remember is that, as the United States entered the twentieth century, TB mortality among the general population had long passed its peak, yet it remained the leading cause of death.

The Twentieth Century

In the United States TB was the leading cause of death from 1900 through 1911 (Figure 3.1). By 1912, fewer deaths were caused by TB than heart disease. In the mid-twentieth century, researchers were suggesting that TB in the United States would be so rare as to constitute a medical curiosity by the beginning of the twenty-first century. In the United States the number of deaths from all forms of TB fell from 194.4 per 100,000 population in 1900 to 0.7 per 100,000 population in 1985. More recently, however, there has been a disturbing resurgence of TB in certain regions of the country. Increased concern has inspired calls for its elimination in the United States by the year 2010.

In 1900 the death rate from pulmonary TB was 173 deaths per 100,000 people. Deaths from pulmonary TB, therefore, accounted for 89 percent of total deaths from the disease reported in the Death Registration Area, which included about 41 percent of the total population. For undetermined reasons, the percentage of deaths from pulmonary TB declined annually until 1913. In 1913 the death rate from all forms of TB was about 144 per 100,000, and the death rate from pulmonary TB was 119 per 100,000. At this point the pulmonary TB death rate was just under 83 percent of that for all forms of the disease. Subsequently, the pulmonary TB death rate increased over the next 20 years, reaching 90 percent of deaths from TB in 1933. Until

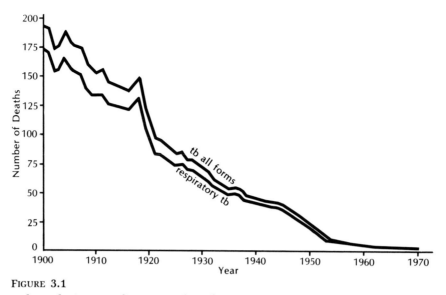

FIGURE **3.1**
Tuberculosis Mortality Rates (Deaths per 100,000 population), 1900–1970

recently, the annual number of deaths from pulmonary TB accounted for between 90 and 94 percent of the total number of deaths from TB.

Geographic Patterns in Mortality Rates

1935. In 1935, the first year for which data are available for each state, the average mortality rate from respiratory TB was 50 deaths per 100,000 population (Figure 3.2). Particularly notable was the concentration of high TB mortality rates in the southwestern United States. Among these states, Arizona stood out, with a mortality rate of 214 deaths per 100,000 people. As for respiratory TB, mortality rates between 96 and 99 per 100,000 were found in the neighboring states of Nevada and New Mexico. The much higher than average death rates in these states were principally the result of TB among the large numbers of Native Americans, most of whom live on reservations or in the larger cities in substandard housing and with inadequate diet, health, and medical care.

Other states with higher-than-average death rates from respiratory TB included Texas, Louisiana, Mississippi, Tennessee, Kentucky, and Virginia. In these states, high death rates from TB were found principally among the poorest populations regardless of race, but the large numbers of poor among the black populations were especially prone to TB infection and mortality. Again, the lack of adequate nutritional levels and adequate care for the poor contributed to especially high death rates among these populations.

Lower-than-national-average rates of between 15 and 35 deaths from respiratory TB per 100,000 people were concentrated in midwestern states. Especially notable was the cluster of states including Wisconsin, Minnesota, Iowa, North Dakota, South Dakota, Nebraska, and Kansas. These states were very rural in character, as are Wyoming, Idaho, and Utah—other states with lower-than-average death rates from respiratory TB.

1945. By 1945, the national average death rate from respiratory TB was 37 deaths per 100,000 people (Figure 3.3). With certain limited exceptions, the 1945 pattern of mortality rates from respiratory TB was remarkably similar to that observed in 1935. Especially notable was the similarity in the distribution of states with lower-than-average death rates, that is, between 11 and 24 deaths per 100,000 people. The only variation is that Maine was in the average range of states, which had between 28 and 45 respiratory TB deaths per 100,000 people. Otherwise the states with low mortality rates again were concentrated in the upper Midwest and the West.

In 1945, as in 1935, Arizona remained in a class by itself, with 200 respiratory TB deaths per 100,000 people. Living conditions among Native Americans and to a lesser extent among the increasing numbers of Mexican Americans who were migrating to Arizona again accounted for the exceptionally high rates. The pattern of states with very high mortality rates in 1945 differed from the pattern 10 years earlier. Very high rates were found, again, in Nevada and New Mexico. California, Texas, Louisiana, Alabama, and Virginia—

states which had had very high death rates from respiratory TB in 1935—by 1945 had rates closer to the lower national average.

1950. By 1950, the national average death rate from respiratory TB had decreased to 21 deaths per 100,000 people (Figure 3.4). The pattern remained similar to that of 1945, as Arizona had an exceptionally high death rate of 189 per 100,000 people and neighboring New Mexico had a rate of 60 deaths. Kentucky, Tennessee, and Maryland, with death rates between 32 and 37 per 100,000 people, retained rates higher than the national average. Arkansas also had a relatively high death rate from respiratory TB.

1960. The national average death rate from TB continued to decline after 1950 (Figure 3.5). In 1960 only 6 persons died from respiratory TB for every 100,000 people in the United States. Despite this decline, several states remained consistent in their much higher than average TB mortality rate. Again, these included Arizona, Arkansas, Kentucky, and Tennessee, with much reduced rates of between 9.4 and 11.0 deaths per 100,000. Higher-than-average death rates in 1960, from 6.9 to 8.5, were also evident in Oklahoma, Missouri, Louisiana, and Alabama. Added to this group in 1960 were a cluster of states in the Northeast, including New York, Rhode Island, and Pennsylvania. Since 1935, Maryland has consistently fallen into the group of states with higher-than-average death rates from respiratory TB.

1985–1989. As mentioned earlier, by 1985 the national average mortality from respiratory TB had declined to 0.7 deaths per 100,000 people. With such a low rate, a more useful comparison between states can be made on the basis of total case rates per 100,000 people, rather than on the basis of death rates. Between 1963 and 1986, the number of reported cases of pulmonary TB declined, on average, 5.0 percent per year. TB case rates per 100,000 population for 1985 for each state are presented in Figure 3.6. These data show that South Carolina, Hawaii, and Alaska had exceptionally high case rates (between 17 and 21 per 100,000 people). Also, the southeastern states combined with Arkansas and Texas to form a solid core of states with between 12 and 15 TB cases per 100,000 persons—again higher than the national average. A higher incidence of TB among poor minorities—especially Hispanics, blacks, Haitians, and Asians—most likely accounted for the higher case rates in these states. In the northern tier of states, only New York had a state average higher than that of the nation. Again, large concentrations of poor and newly arrived ethnic minorities living in New York City and its environs, including large numbers of Haitians, Puerto Ri-

cans, and Asians, probably accounted for this situation.

Very low TB case rates of fewer than 4 per 100,000 persons were found consistently among states of the upper Midwest. With the exceptions of South Dakota and Montana, from Wisconsin westward to Idaho and from North Dakota and Minnesota south to Utah, Colorado, and Kansas, there was a solid block of states with the lowest TB case rates in the country. New Hampshire and Vermont in the upper Northeast also had very low TB case rates.

In 1985, on average, for every case of TB among whites there were 5.2 cases among nonwhites (Figure 3.7). More specifically, the rate among Hispanics was 18 per 100,000 people, compared to 4.5 per 100,000 among the non-Hispanic white population. Nationally, 48 percent of TB cases occurred among nonwhites, 38 percent among non-Hispanic whites, and 14 percent among Hispanics. By 1989, the overall TB case rate in the United States had increased to 9.5 per 100,000 people. However, among foreign-born persons arriving in the United States, the case rate was 124 per 100,000 people, or 13 times as high as among the resident population. Further, between 1986 and 1989, 22 percent of all reported TB cases occurred in the foreign-born population. The association between race and ethnicity in TB case rates is further illustrated in Figure 3.8, which depicts the geographic distribution of nonwhite and white TB case rates. In California, Texas, and New York, higher-than-average TB rates occurred principally among Hispanic populations. California reported 40 percent of the cases among Hispanics; Texas, 23 percent; and New York, 13 percent.

Among blacks, the incidence rate of TB was 27 per 100,000 in 1985. The relative risk of TB among black males was 6.2 times higher than that of white males; among black females the risk for TB was 5.1 times higher than that of white females. The majority of TB cases in blacks occurred in New York, Florida, Georgia, Illinois, Texas, South Carolina, North Carolina, New Jersey, and Alabama. It has been suspected for some time that blacks may be more susceptible to infection by the TB bacterium than whites. Results from a recent large-scale study of integrated nursing homes were reported in the *New England Journal of Medicine*. These results suggest that blacks are twice as likely to be infected with the TB bacterium as are whites living in the same exposure conditions. Though it is incredibly difficult to separate out environmental causes that might account for racial differences, there may be some genetic predisposition to TB infection among certain populations.

Among Native Americans and Alaskan Natives, the incidence rate was 25 per 100,000, 4.4 times the rate for the white population. Native Americans and Alaskan Natives accounted for large proportions of reported

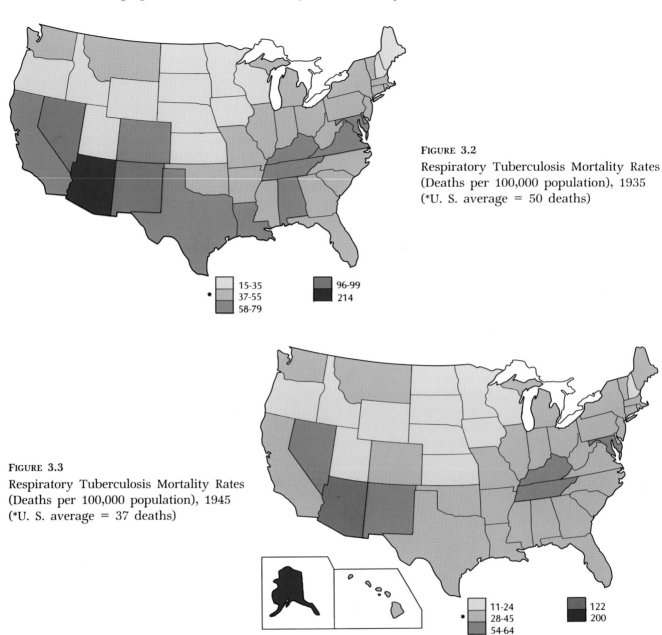

FIGURE 3.2
Respiratory Tuberculosis Mortality Rates
(Deaths per 100,000 population), 1935
(*U. S. average = 50 deaths)

	15-35	96-99
*	37-55	214
	58-79	

FIGURE 3.3
Respiratory Tuberculosis Mortality Rates
(Deaths per 100,000 population), 1945
(*U. S. average = 37 deaths)

	11-24	122
*	28-45	200
	54-64	

TB cases in Alaska and South Dakota. The high rates of morbidity and mortality from TB observed among Native Americans at the end of the last century have been attributed to increased contact with the white civilization. This is also believed to be the case in Alaska, where the morbidity rates from TB in the early 1950s were the highest ever reported in the medical literature. Again, perhaps an increased predispostion to TB infection may be present due to a relatively short period of contact with the disease.

Asians and Pacific Islanders in the United States, however, had the highest TB incidence rates. In 1985 the rate for these groups was about 50 per 100,000 persons. The largest number of cases occurred in Califor-

nia, Hawaii, New York, Texas, and Illinois. However, 94 percent of the cases were foreign-born, predominantly from Laos, Vietnam, the Philippines, Korea, and China.

Geography of Urban Tuberculosis

Traditionally, TB has been identified with the city. It has long been recognized that early industrialization and overcrowding of cities produced epidemics of tuberculosis by bringing together large numbers of susceptible people and promoting transmission of the tubercle bacillus. The experience of England's large in-

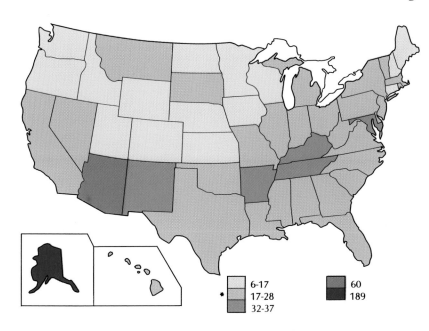

FIGURE 3.4
Respiratory Tuberculosis Mortality Rates
(Deaths per 100,000 population), 1950
(*U. S. average = 21 deaths)

6-17	60
17-28	189
32-37	

FIGURE 3.5
Respiratory Tuberculosis Mortality Rates
(Deaths per 100,000 population), 1960
(*U. S. average = 5.6 deaths)

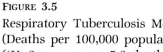

1.6-3.3	6.9-8.5
3.6-5.0	9.4-11.0
5.2-6.1	

dustrialized cities was repeated in the United States. Exceptionally high mortality rates occurred among poor and minority groups concentrated in the crowded sections of the large and industrial cities. Today, higher-than-average case rates for TB also occur in cities among lower-income and minority populations. There are significant geographic variations in the higher-than-average TB case rates by race and ethnicity in all U.S. cities that have at least 250,000 residents, as illustrated in Figure 3.9.

Generally, the racial composition of higher-than-average TB case rates is concentrated among nonwhite populations in cities of the eastern third of the United States. These cities include Boston, New York,

Washington, D.C., Detroit, Chicago, and Atlanta. In Miami and San Francisco, TB is concentrated among nonwhite and Hispanic populations. In Texas, New Mexico, and Arizona, higher-than-average TB case rates are found principally among Hispanics in cities such as Houston, San Antonio, El Paso, Albuquerque, and Tucson.

Among cities in the United States, in 1985 the TB case rate ranged from a low of 2 per 100,000 to a high of 48 per 100,000. As illustrated in Figure 3.9, generally the lowest TB case rates were found in midwestern cities. While there were some exceptions, rates between 2 and 11 cases per 100,000 were found in cities such as Columbus and Toledo, Indianapolis,

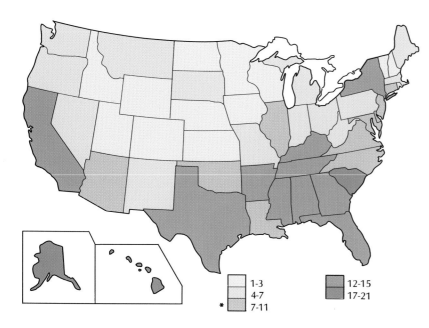

FIGURE 3.6
Tuberculosis Rates (Cases per 100,000 population), 1985 (*U. S. average = 9.3 cases)

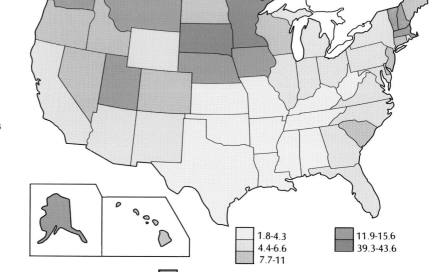

FIGURE 3.7
Tuberculosis Rates among Non-Whites (Cases per 100,000 population), 1985

Kansas City, Minneapolis-Saint Paul, Denver, and Albuquerque. Among cities with low TB case rates, however, there was a geographic difference in the distribution of concentration of higher-than-average case rates, which were found among non-Hispanic white populations in Toledo, Indianapolis, Tulsa and Oklahoma City, and in Omaha. Case rates were higher than average among nonwhites in Columbus; Kansas City; and Colorado Springs. Interestingly, higher-than-average case rates occurred among nonwhites in Saint Paul, while in its twin city of Minneapolis, higher-than-average case rates occurred among nonwhites and non-Hispanic whites.

The highest TB case rates among cities with more than 250,000 people occurred in Atlanta, Miami, and San Francisco. In these cities, case rates ranged from 42 to 48 per 100,000 population. In Atlanta the higher-than-average case rates occurred predominantly among nonwhites, while in San Francisco and Miami they were concentrated among nonwhites and Hispanics.

Conclusion

Today, TB in the United States remains a relatively insignificant health threat, in comparison to its severity

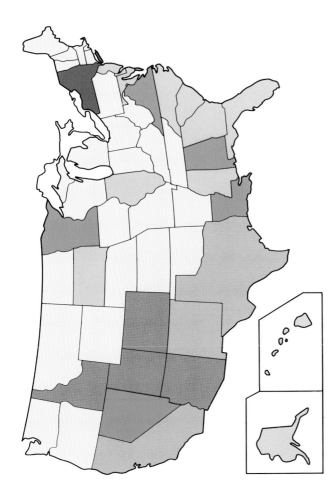

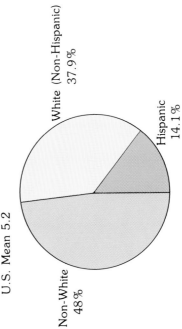

Colors represent higher than average
percent of cases by race and ethnicity.

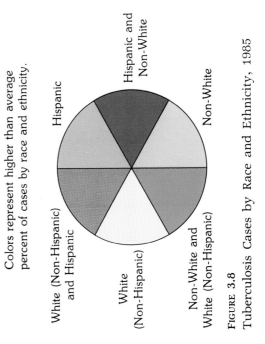

Hispanic

Hispanic and
Non-White

White (Non-Hispanic)
and Hispanic

White
(Non-Hispanic)

Non-White and
White (Non-Hispanic)

Non-White

Average percent of cases by race and
ethnicity based on U.S. mean
U.S. Mean 5.2

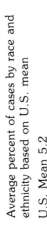

White (Non-Hispanic)
37.9%

Hispanic
14.1%

Non-White
48%

FIGURE 3.8
Tuberculosis Cases by Race and Ethnicity, 1985

31

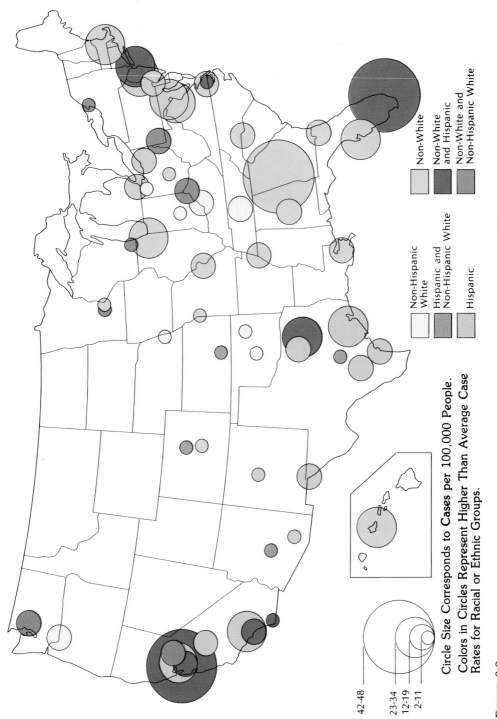

Non-Hispanic
White

Hispanic and
Non-Hispanic White

Hispanic

Non-White

Non-White
and Hispanic

Non-White and
Non-Hispanic White

Circle Size Corresponds to Cases per 100,000 People.

Colors in Circles Represent Higher Than Average Case
Rates for Racial or Ethnic Groups.

42-48
23-34
12-19
2-11

FIGURE 3.9
Urban Tuberculosis Cases, 1985

in the early part of the twentieth century. What is disturbing, however, is that the steady decline experienced over the past decades has been arrested. By and large, the problem is the occurrence of TB among large numbers of immigrants from Asia, the Pacific Islands, and the Caribbean, as well as among Hispanics, blacks, Native Americans, and Alaskan Natives. The government has recently published a plan for eliminating TB from the United States by the year 2010. This plan focuses on increased testing for TB among prospective immigrants to the United States to prevent their entry and on provision of treatment and screening for TB. Of particular concern is the resurgence of TB among acquired immune deficiency syndrome (AIDS) victims. In these cases, most frequently, the TB is not a new infection but an old infection which recurs because of a depleted immune system resulting from human immunodeficiency virus (HIV) infection. Additionally disturbing is the statement of leading health scientists that the "new" TB may be drug-resistant. In early 1991 at least 13 states reported one drug-resistant case of TB. This development is especially important because the TB bacillus is the only opportunistic infection that can be spread from people infected with HIV to others who are not infected.

"THE CAPTAIN OF ALL THESE MEN OF DEATH" has certainly been reduced in rank as a major killer disease in the United States during the twentieth century. However, the future of the disease remains uncertain, as old infections are revitalized under the influence of the Human Immunodeficiency Virus; as more immigrants bring active TB with them; as people continue to live in unhealthy settings; and as a small but growing and widely scattered number of TB cases are found to be resistant to current antibiotic medicines.

INFLUENZA

Influenza, often accompanied by pneumonia, is one of the ten leading causes of death in the United States. Historically, descriptions of epidemics that are probably due to influenza have included descriptions of how and when the disease spread from one place to another. It is not difficult to reconstruct origin and diffusion pathways of influenza epidemics during the twentieth century in the United States. Such information helps epidemiologists to understand the behavior of the disease as it spreads from individual to individual and from city to city. As discussed below, the agent that causes influenza was not discovered in its true form until the early 1930s, even though people suspected that a virus carried the disease earlier in the twentieth century and in previous centuries. Therefore, descriptions of influenza epidemics prior to the twentieth century rely heavily on descriptions of the disease and symptoms that appear to be similar to those now known to cause influenza. The best accounts of influenza epidemics prior to the twentieth century are found in European records. Most of these accounts show how the disease appears to have spread in relation to transportation accessibility and susceptible numbers of people. Diffusion of the first modern-day forms of influenza probably took place when the European railroad network had been completed after the Industrial Revolution and near the end of the nineteenth century, in what was known as the *"influenza epidemic of 1889–1892."* This form of influenza also spread to the United States in 1889.

Geography and Influenza Genetics

Influenza is transferred from one person to another by the respiratory route, probably via moisture droplets. The incubation period is relatively short, from 24 to 72 hours, and transmission can be quite rapid, especially if one of the more virulent forms of influenza is involved. New and novel strains of the disease are often more virulent than previous ones, but this is not always the case. In temperate latitudes such as the United States and Europe, epidemics usually occur during the winter, although late-summer outbreaks are known. It is also of interest that northern and southern hemispheres often experience influenza epidemics 6 months apart, a pattern that is especially clear after the introduction of a new strain of the disease. The reason for this transequatorial swing is probably seasonal, since influenza does appear to be a wintertime disease. Cold, dry air seems to favor the spread of the virus, probably because people tend to congregate inside more during cold weather. In addition, school-year calendars also seem to coincide with the timing of influenza outbreaks. Sometimes students returning to school from vacation periods bring influenza epidemics with them. Seasonality of the disease is much less evident in the tropics, although when a new strain is introduced, it will spread very fast during particularly dry seasons.

Many epidemiologists believe that conditions for the propagation of new worldwide forms of influenza appear to be particularly favorable in central Asia and the western parts of China. Historically, people of many cultures have often assumed that new forms of influenza, and other serious diseases for that matter, were brought by strangers or people other than themselves. Many European accounts of influenza during the nineteenth century, for example, claim that epidemics originated in central Asia or China. However, there are also ethnocentrically based terms for the disease, such as "French sweat," "Englishman's disease," and "Scottish rant." Even during the twentieth century, we have adopted such labels as "Spanish influenza," "Asian flu," "Hong Kong flu," and "Russian flu." Actually, specific geographic origins of most influenza epidemics are not very well known, and we can only speculate about broad general regions of the world because by the time pandemics (worldwide epidemics) are well established, thousands of persons have already been infected. It is then necessary to do geographical backtracking to determine points of origin of specific diseases, and pinpointing the zones of actual origin is often quite difficult. Many epidemics that have swept through the United States do seem to have started in other parts of the world. Epidemics that may have originated on the U.S. continent seem to have been caused by prevailing strains of the disease rather than by the newly emerging types of viruses that are more likely to start pandemics.

The actual influenza virus has 8 separate strains of ribonucleic acid (RNA) for its hereditary material. Like most viruses, it can reproduce only within the cells of a higher organism. When a cell is simultaneously infected with two different varieties of the virus, the 16 RNA segments can recombine to produce progeny with traits from both of the parent strains. This unusual system gives the flu virus enormous flexibility, enabling it to evolve into new strains and to withstand hosts' immunological defenses. Two of the eight viral genes code form protein-sugar complexes on the outer coat of the virus. These surface molecules, hemagglutinin (H) and neuraminidase (N), are antigens which can stimulate the host immune system to make antibodies against the infecting virus. Thirteen different H and six N subtypes have been discovered in birds and mammals. New human strains may originate in the cells of wild and domestic animals. Subtypes H1, H2, H3, N1, and N2 are known to have caused human influenza. Major "shifts" in the virus, that is, the appearance of new HN or N antigens, have taken place probably in 1889, 1918, 1957, 1968, and 1977, each time causing a pandemic. Smaller genetic changes in the structure of H and N molecules can take place almost constantly. This accumulation of small mutations is known as "drift," and it also helps the virus to evade host defenses, although usually not as completely as in the case of totally new subtypes. Between pandemics, drifting strains continue to circulate and may, as the H1N1 variance of 1928–1929 and 1947–1948, cause serious epidemics. There is also some evidence that only a limited number of H and N subtypes can produce epidemics. For example, immunological studies of elderly survivors of the 1889–1892 pandemic suggest that it was caused by a virus with an H antigen very similar to that of the 1957 virus. Several postulated relationships thus exist. For example, the 1889–1892 pandemic may have recycled in 1957–1958 as Asian flu, as suggested in Figure 3.10, and may have been replaced in 1968 by H3N2. In addition, there is some reason to believe that a recycled form of H3N2 from early in the nineteenth century eventually reappeared in 1968–

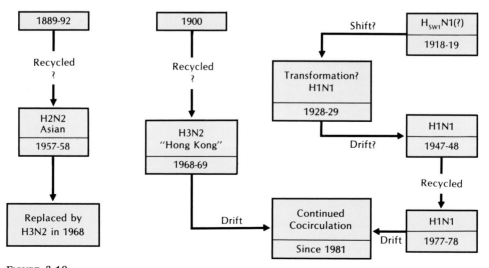

FIGURE 3.10
Influenza Genetics

1969 and has continued to circulate since the early 1980s, along with another strain. A third possible sequence of events includes the transformation of swine flu (a form of influenza which occurs in hogs and is closely related to human influenza), HSW1N1, in 1918–1919, and then a retransformation in 1928–1929, which drifted to the 1947–1948 H1N1 strain that recycled in the late 1970s and was sometimes known as "Russian flu." The H1N1 strain now circulates with an earlier form of Hong Kong flu, thus making the mapping of influenza epidemics difficult, but not impossible.

International Dimensions of the 1918–1919 Pandemic

The twentieth-century influenza diffusion patterns that have affected the United States fall into two main categories—forms that appear to have invaded the country from abroad and forms that have originated deep within the interior of the North American continent. Forms from abroad are easier to identify because they are normally first noticed in seaports. It is common for densely settled parts of the northeastern United States and California to emerge early as epidemic influenza areas. The relationship between the virulence of the influenza virus and geographic spread can then be understood by the speed at which numbers of cases increase over time. For example, if a virus is especially potent and there are only small numbers of immune people, the disease will spread rapidly through metropolitan regions and will sometimes leapfrog from one large population center to another, while simultaneously spreading into surrounding hinterlands. This effect can be determined in a fairly systematic manner as smaller and smaller areas within an urban hierarchy become centers for local diffusion. Less virulent strains of extraneous origin spread more slowly, and hierarchical patterns of diffusion are much less pronounced, or at least more difficult to identify. Diffusion patterns during epidemics of previously prevalent strains differ from those created by new strains because, more often than not, they spread from epicenters in interior parts of the country.

The first twentieth-century influenza pandemic coincided with the end of World War I. Tens of millions of people died worldwide from influenza and its complications. More than half a million Americans perished in the devastating wave which swept the nation from September 1918 to March 1919. The pandemic took the form of two and possibly three distinct temporal waves. Had these waves occurred from 2 to 3 years apart, they might have been considered separate epidemics.

The first wave has been identified as having taken place in the spring of 1918. Many accounts indicate that it began in the midwestern part of the United States (note the pattern in Figure 3.11). The earliest record outbreak seems to have occurred among U.S. army recruits at training camps in central Kansas, where an epidemic began in early March of 1918. Influenza spread to military training installations in several midwestern and southeastern states by the end of March. During April, the virus became more widely diffused across the country and began to affect civilians as well as military populations.

Reconstruction of the epidemic indicates that the influenza reached France aboard American troop ships in April 1918 and spread quickly to the front in that war-torn country. The disease also seems to have spread to Spain by May; the term "Spanish flu" originated because newspaper accounts from an uncensored country were not made available. It had already spread to China by May 1918, and by June, it had spread into Central America and South America, as well as the Philippines and India. Early incidence of the influenza in China was probably caused by trans-Pacific transport from the United States, although there may have been one or two local outbreaks of another virus. There is also no evidence that clearly indicates that the 1918 first wave was brought to North America from China and then on to France by Chinese laborers making their way to the western front.

During July and August of 1918, there was a lull in influenza activity due to seasonal factors, an event not uncommon in influenza epidemics. The first wave seems to have spread to some of the more urbanized parts of the world by late summer. Overall mortality rates were low, by contrast to what happened later, but in some places there seem to have been disproportionately higher mortality rates among young adults in both military and civilian populations. This information is important because it suggests that there was probably a close relationship between the spring virus and the more deadly strain that covered the world so rapidly later that year.

The second wave, or fall strain, which was more lethal and was likely to be accompanied by bacterial pneumonias, seems to have surfaced in early August, perhaps as a genetic mutation or recombination. The first reports were from France, and the disease spread rapidly from France to Spain and down to western Africa during August 1918. By September, this much more deadly European strain was well established in the northeastern part of the United States, in the Pacific Northwest, in southern California, and in the U.S. Gulf Coast area, as well as in Brazil, Argentina, western Africa, South Africa, parts of India, China, Japan, and most of Western Europe (note the pattern in Figure 3.12. As this pandemic of influenza continued to

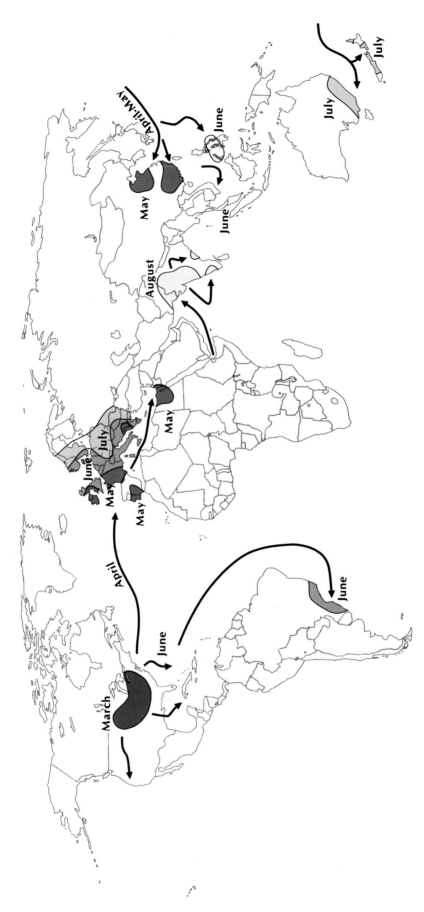

FIGURE 3.11
Worldwide Diffusion of Influenza: First Wave, Spring 1918

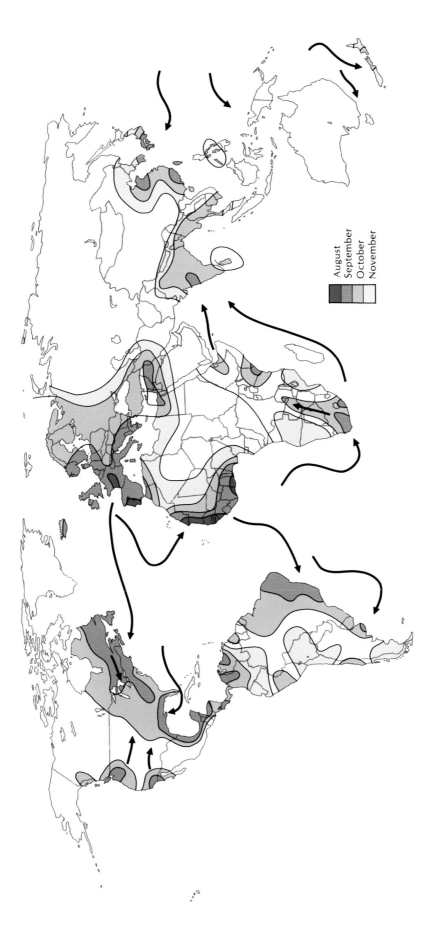

FIGURE 3.12
Worldwide Diffusion of Influenza: Second Wave, Autumn 1918

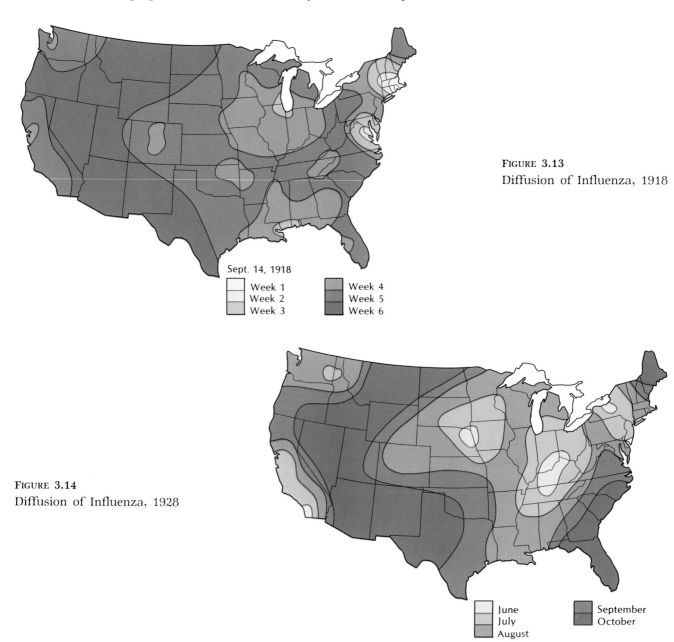

FIGURE 3.13
Diffusion of Influenza, 1918

Sept. 14, 1918
Week 1
Week 2
Week 3
Week 4
Week 5
Week 6

FIGURE 3.14
Diffusion of Influenza, 1928

June
July
August
September
October

spread through more settled parts of the world during October and November 1918, the death toll became enormous; precise mortality totals may never be known because of incompleteness of reporting and inaccuracy of diagnoses in different parts of the world. Further confusion arose because assigning the cause of death was often difficult due to the accompanying pneumonia. There were also many deaths attributed to pneumonia, cardiovascular disease, diabetes, and other diseases that might have been directly or indirectly related to the pandemic of influenza.

The first major reports of influenza in the United States during the second wave were from New England. Influenza reached Boston from France in late August 1918 and appeared right after that in Washing-

ton, D.C. (see the pattern in Figure 3.13). The epidemic then leapfrogged to Chicago and spread from that metropolis into the country's agricultural heartland in a radial fashion. Troops returning from France also brought influenza to many military bases in the Southeast, which in turn acted as diffusion centers for that part of the country. Since the South at that time was mostly rural, no single city reported the substantial numbers of cases that showed up in parts of the Northeast. The epidemic also spread rapidly to western parts of the country from Pacific seaports.

Dense concentrations of people in industrial centers during that time in U.S. history contributed to the severity and rapid spread of the epidemic in the more urbanized parts of the country. Under normal circum-

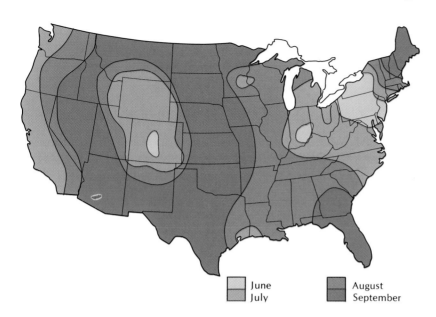

FIGURE 3.15
Diffusion of Influenza, 1947

June
July

August
September

FIGURE 3.16
Diffusion of Influenza, 1977–1978

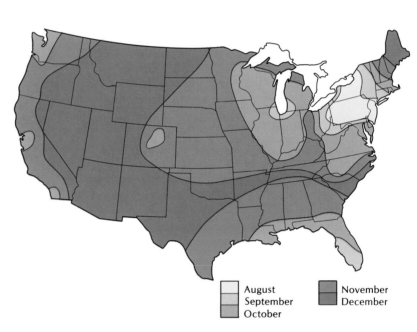

August
September
October

November
December

stances, influenza epidemics take their heaviest toll among the elderly, who are particularly vulnerable to secondary pneumonia because immune systems often weaken with age. The next most affected group is the very young. These age groups have been at greatest risk in every influenza epidemic since at least the year 1700. There was a crucial difference in the 1918–1919 pandemic, however, in that much higher than expected mortality rates occurred among the 20-to-40-year-old group as well as among the very young and the elderly. The exact reason why so many young adults were devastated during this pandemic remains a mystery, and subsequent patterns of influenza epidemics within the United States have shown no repetition of this pattern.

Influenza in the 1920s

After the major pandemic of 1918–1919, there were less serious outbreaks of influenza as well as so-called mini-epidemics through the early 1920s, but none were so severe as the second wave of 1918. The strain of virus that caused the 1918 second wave probably transformed into less virulent H1N1 types during the late 1920s. A contrasting pattern of influenza diffusion, for example, can be seen when patterns of spread during the autumn of 1928 are identified (note Figure 3.14). The outbreak during the fall of 1928 led to the epidemic of 1928–1929, and what we now consider "normal" patterns of death rates occurred among the elderly and the very young. Furthermore, the geographic spread of the 1928–1929 epidemic took the form of outbreaks within epicenters of the interior United States and, with the exception of California, not in coastal areas. Such a pattern indicates an endemic, or established, pattern as opposed to one with external origins. The epidemic of 1928–1929 was also characterized by much slower patterns of geographic spread, another indication that the virus was different from the more virulent form of the second wave of 1918. Mild forms of the 1928–1929 strain seem to have continued to circulate within the U.S. population during the 1940s.

Geographic Patterns in Mortality Rates

The 1930s and the 1940s. There were more deaths from influenza and pneumonia during almost every winter of the Great Depression than in subsequent decades. These deaths may have been a reflection of economic conditions during those times, when (as shown in other parts of this atlas) death rates were very high in the United States in general. There was a minor epidemic of influenza during the height of World War II. Epidemics do seem to go hand in hand with wars, and the spread of many kinds of diseases is often inevitable, due to major viral shifts. The most significant event in influenza history during the 1930s was the discovery of the actual influenza virus in both British and American laboratories. Subsequent laboratory isolations of viruses showed that strains similar to the 1928–1929 virus were still active during the Depression and World War II. Medical research also eventually led to the development of influenza vaccines during the 1940s.

To the disappointment and surprise of many researchers, however, a vaccine developed during the mid-1940s seemed to provide little immunity to a virus that caused another major epidemic during the 1947–1948 winter. The failure of this newly developed vaccine to halt the spread of influenza might have been due to the fact that a slightly different strain of the disease had surfaced. Fortunately, the epidemic that started spreading in the United States during the fall of 1947 was not the lethal brand of influenza that had surfaced after World War I. Its rate of progression (the pattern is shown in Figure 3.15) was thus measured in months rather than weeks. Contemporary influenza research indicates that the epidemic was not a surprise. It had begun in July in the urban Northeast. Early epicenters subsequently showed up on the West Coast, in the Gulf Coast area, in central Colorado, in Minneapolis-Saint Paul, and in the Ohio Valley. Such scattered early reporting suggests that a variant of this modified strain may have entered the United States in the spring of 1947 and spread slowly during the summer, a time of minimal influenza activity. It does seem clear that the epidemic did not originate in the United States, because large sections of the Northeast were reporting higher-than-normal numbers of influenza deaths as early as July 1947. By August, the disease had spread into the remainder of New England, the upper Midwest, and the Southeast. The outbreaks in other parts of the country also served as centers for diffusion of the disease into the interior parts of the country. There were also European reports of a similar strain of influenza virus at that time, and the 1947 strain appears to have been a dominant type that continued to show up throughout the world for another decade or so.

The 1950s, the 1960s, and the 1970s. At approximately 10-year intervals, beginning in 1947, outbreaks occurred in the late 1950s, in the late 1960s, and in the late 1970s. The strains were not all the same. In 1957, a pandemic of Asian flu (H2N2) spread outward from Asia during the fall. During the winter of 1957–1958, patterns of spatial diffusion were drastically different from previous patterns. The pandemic, which probably started in China, initially reached the United States on the West Coast. It then spread to the East, probably during the late summer and early autumn of 1957. The strain also seems to have spread into the United States from the Gulf Coast area, as in some previous pandemics. In this pandemic, unlike the great pandemic of 1918, there was very little early diffusion from urban to rural places within the United States. Instead, the west-to-east spread was well documented by the U.S. Public Health Service. It was only after the epidemic had spread across the country from west to east during the late summer and early fall of 1957 that regional patterns of radial diffusion could be discerned.

Similarly, in 1968, the Hong Kong (H3N2) strain originated in Asia. As in 1957, there was a very broad pattern of west-to-east diffusion of the disease during the summer and early fall; however, it is impossible to identify well-defined patterns of spread during this pandemic. There was also an outbreak of a prevailing strain of influenza during the spring of 1967, and there may have been some genetic "mixing" of a couple of strains during the summer of 1968, a situation that would tend to dampen the effects of a single shift in genetic makeup of the virus. After the early outbreaks of the newer strain in July and August of 1968, influenza then began to spread outward from multiple epicenters within the United States.

Many epidemiologists who had closely monitored both mild and severe influenza pandemics feared that there might be a major pandemic of influenza during the late 1970s. Many believed that another catastrophe

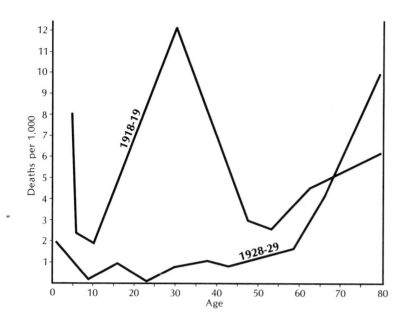

FIGURE 3.17
Influenza Mortality Age Structure
Comparisons, 1918–1919 and 1928–1929

similar to the deadly pandemic of 1918 would occur, and some of these suspicions were confirmed by the emergence of a form of swine flu that appeared early in 1976. This circumstance led to a controversial swine flu inoculation program during the autumn of 1976, but a "new" strain of influenza nonetheless seems to have appeared in China or central Asia early in 1977 and entered the United States during the late summer or early autumn. During the autumn of 1977, influenza spread in patterns very similar to those of 1918 and 1947, although at a pace more similar to that of the epidemic of the 1940s than to that of the earlier pandemic (the pattern is shown in Figure 3.16). As in 1947, the first major outbreaks were in the densely populated northeastern parts of the country. The 1977 virus was nearly identical to the one that had caused the epidemic 30 years earlier, rather than being the kind of strain that had appeared in 1957 and 1968. After the initial northeastern outbreaks, nodes for subsequent spread of the disease popped up in southern Florida, the greater Chicago metropolitan area, Denver, and parts of the West Coast. While the 1947–1948 and 1977–1978 diffusion patterns were very similar, increased mortality in Florida during the 1970s epidemic was indicative of that state's growth as a retirement area during the late twentieth century.

The 1980s and Beyond. Influenza geography during the 1980s in the United States became even more complicated because there was substantial comingling between the 1977–1978 strain and the 1968 strain. Many things can be learned by examining the various pat-

terns of influenza diffusion within the United States. The most important aspect of such studies is that even though many innovations have been made in transportation technologies during this century, epidemics of infectious diseases still tend to gravitate toward large cities where there are substantial pools of susceptible populations. Epidemics thus move in a hierarchical pattern from larger to smaller places, and there is regional spreading from major centers to surrounding hinterlands. In addition, as the number of cities becomes larger, forming many more nodes for diffusion, epidemics spread in a similar fashion. The nature of the U.S. urban system is thus a key factor in understanding disease diffusion.

Examination of such disease information also tells us something about different types of epidemics. For example, the common forms of influenza mortality occur among the elderly and, to some extent, among the very young. As previously mentioned, the one exception was the pandemic of 1918–1919, which also affected a large proportion of the 20-to-40-year-old group (note the comparison in Figure 3.17). It is thus very important to examine rates of infection among various age groups carefully so as to determine pathways of spread, since there are different concentrations of age cohorts within various parts of the United States. The importance of the demographic geography of areas can also be seen. For example, if there are heavier concentrations of elderly people in both central cities and rural areas, then such locations can be expected to be more heavily impacted during influenza epidemics.

4

Chronic Disease Mortality: An Overview

In the late 1980s, chronic diseases were the dominant underlying diagnoses in the deaths of more than 1 million people in the United States each year. In 1986, chronic diseases (stroke, coronary heart disease, diabetes, chronic obstructive pulmonary disease, lung cancer, female breast cancer, cervical cancer, colorectal cancer, and chronic liver disease including cirrhosis) accounted for 52 percent of deaths (1.1 million). The overall age-adjusted mortality rate for these nine chronic diseases was 458 deaths per 100,000 Americans.

A large majority of deaths from chronic diseases are preventable. Such behaviors and conditions as cigarette smoking, hypertension, obesity, high cholesterol levels, sedentary lifestyle, heavy consumption of alcohol, and failure to take advantage of or not having access to screening techniques such as mammography and Pap smears significantly increase the risk of death from these chronic diseases. Other social and environmental factors which contribute to chronic disease mortality include lack of knowledge of risk factors and lack of access to medical care.

Geographic Variation

In an attempt to assess statistical and geographic variation in the distribution of mortality from the nine leading chronic diseases, the Centers for Disease Control developed and computed combined age-adjusted mortality rates for each state and for the nation. The resulting mortality rates for 1986 illustrate a substantial geographic variation in the death rates from these diseases (Figure 4.1).

As mentioned above, the combined average age-adjusted mortality rate for nine chronic diseases was 458 deaths per 100,000 people. The range of the mortality rates was considerable, however. The lowest mortality rate occurred in Hawaii (327 deaths per 100,000) and the highest in Michigan (518 per 100,000).

Of particular geographic significance was a cluster of states with exceptionally high mortality rates for chronic diseases (over 500 deaths per 100,000 population) in the northeast. In 1986, these states were led by Michigan, with the highest age-adjusted rate (518 per 100,000). Michigan was followed by West Virginia (513 per 100,000), New York (509 per 100,000), and Ohio (501 per 100,000). Rhode Island (491 per 100,000) and South Carolina (493 per 100,000) also had exceptionally high mortality rates, as compared to other states.

With the exception of Nevada and Oklahoma, states with higher-than-average mortality rates (ranging from 467 to 482 deaths per 100,000 population) were located in the eastern half of the United States. The geographic locations of these states extended from Maine (475 per 100,000) in the Northeast, through

42

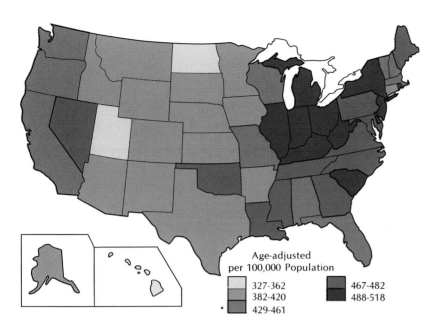

Age-adjusted
per 100,000 Population

327-362   467-482
382-420   488-518
429-461

FIGURE 4.1
Combined Mortality Rates from Nine Chronic Diseases (Deaths per 100,000 population), 1986 (*U.S. mean = 458)

Pennsylvania (479 per 100,000) and Virginia (467 per 100,000), to Mississippi (469 per 100,000) and Louisiana (470 per 100,000) in the Deep South.

Generally, the central one-third of the United States west of the Mississippi River is characterized by below-average mortality rates from the nine chronic diseases. The lowest rates occurred in Utah (362 per 100,000) and North Dakota (361 per 100,000). With only a few exceptions, states from Minnesota (386 per 100,000) westward to Idaho (395 per 100,000) and southward to Texas (398 per 100,000) and Arizona (396 per 100,000) had mortality rates lower than the national average.

Conclusion

Mortality rates from the nine chronic diseases discussed here could be substantially altered by reducing the risk factors which have been strongly implicated in their development and severity. Many health experts conclude that the estimated decline which could be achieved through risk reduction would result in elimination of 26 to 52 percent of the deaths. For the nation this would mean that approximately 524,000 deaths could be avoided annually.

Of the risk factors that have been examined for their contribution to deaths from the nine chronic diseases, the largest reduction, 33 percent, could be achieved by eliminating cigarette smoking. Substantial reductions could be achieved by reducing obesity (24 percent), sedentary lifestyle (23 percent), high cholesterol levels (23 percent), hypertension (21 percent), and diabetes (8 percent). With regard to specific chronic disease mortality reduction, it has been estimated that about 48

percent of the deaths from coronary heart disease, stroke, and chronic obstructive pulmonary diseases could be eliminated by reducing cholesterol levels, obesity, and smoking, respectively.

A reduction of risks and accompanying chronic disease mortality would also have an impact upon the age structure of the population. It is estimated that the average life expectancy would increase from the current average of 74 to 82 years, as states with higher mortality rates from the nine diseases showed lower life expectancies for their populations.

Though there are nonpreventable contributors to mortality for many diseases, analysis indicates that substantial reductions in mortality and increases in life expectancy could be achieved by placing emphasis upon risk factor reduction. Programs that could have substantially impact upon the lives of many individuals and of society in general should be directed at reducing cigarette smoking; and alleviating hypertension, obesity, high cholesterol levels, lack of exercise, and heavy alcohol consumption; and increasing the use of preventive and screening measures. The critical challenge to society, it would seem, is to implement programs based on established knowledge pertaining to these risk factors, to increase awareness and motivation for healthful living, and to assure access to the necessary resources to combat mortality from these chronic diseases. In this area the United States has a considerable distance to go, since a recent survey of states indicated that 45 states and the District of Columbia reported that less than 2 percent of state public health expenditure was allocated for prevention of chronic diseases.

5

Coronary Heart Disease

In 1991 well over 2 million people died in the United States from all causes. About one-third of all these deaths were caused by what is now officially designated "Ischemic heart disease," the most common of the cardiovascular diseases. This cause of death is informally referred to as "coronary heart disease" and has also been referred to as "arteriosclerotic heart disease."

While it may be presumed that coronary heart disease has always affected humans, its identification is of relatively recent origin. Pathologists in the late nineteenth century were aware that the coronary arteries sometimes became blocked, and they drew the connection between this observation and recurrent chest pain. As a concern of the practicing physician, however, it was not until the 1920s that this disease began to assume some importance. We know now that the heart needs a constant flow of blood and this flow is sometimes restricted by fatty deposits in arteries, a condition known as "atherosclerosis." As the blood flows through arteries that are particularly constricted, clots can form, blocking the artery even further. When the flow of blood becomes severely restricted, a myocardial infarction—commonly known as a "heart attack"—can result.

Due in part to the historical significance of and mortality from other acute and infectious diseases such as pneumonia and tuberculosis and also due in part to the relatively short life expectancy at the turn of the century, it was not until 1929 that the international list of causes of death was revised and the magnitude of mortality from heart disease became evident. As recogni-

tion of its importance as a major killer increased, more attention was directed toward this disease, with several subsequent major changes in classification. The initial broad classification as well as the several major reclassifications make it difficult to assess the distribution of coronary heart disease mortality in the United States since 1900. More recent diagnoses are not comparable to those of the 1920s and 1930s, and a meaningful time line for coronary heart disease probably goes back only to 1940 at the earliest.

It is known that from 1940 through 1969 the crude death rate from heart disease increased almost 50 percent. The increase was also observed in age-adjusted rates. From 1940 through 1960 the age-adjusted death rate, which takes into account the aging population, increased almost 27 percent. There was no increase among white women. The increase was more than 48 percent among nonwhite men, and more than 34 percent among nonwhite women. These increases were probably due at least in part to an increase in the number of physicians trained to recognize the disease. Another part was a secondary result of the greater control of infectious diseases, which led to an increasing proportion of people living to older ages, when they are more vulnerable to coronary heart disease mortality. However, a large part of the rise in heart disease mortality unquestionably was due to a real increase in the force of mortality from this cause.

As a result, the proportion of deaths ascribed to coronary heart disease also rose. It has been estimated that in 1900 approximately 100,000 deaths, or 8 percent of all deaths that year, were the result of heart diseases. This number was surpassed by both pneumonia and tuberculosis. In 1910 heart diseases (147,000), pneumonia (131,000), and tuberculosis (142,000) each accounted for about 11 percent of all deaths. By 1940, about 272,000 deaths, or 21 percent of the total number of deaths in the nation, were ascribed to coronary disease, whereas pneumonia accounted for only 5 percent and tuberculosis for only 4 percent. In 1950 about 31 percent of deaths, or about 350,000 deaths, resulted from coronary heart disease. By 1960, coronary heart disease was responsible for 546,000 deaths, or about 40 percent of all deaths in the United States. In 1986 coronary heart disease accounted for about 600,000 deaths, or 28 percent of all deaths. In 1990 the estimated number of deaths from coronary heart disease was still well over 500,000. However, over the past 30 years something very interesting has happened in the United States.

It appears that mortality from coronary heart disease peaked in the mid-1960s and since then has steadily decreased. Between 1960 and 1967 the death rate for white men changed very little. Age-adjusted coronary death rates for nonwhite men and women appear to have essentially leveled off by 1962, and rates for white women have remained relatively stable since 1940. By 1985, the age-adjusted coronary heart disease death rate had decreased to about 70 percent of the 1950 rate. The decline occurred among males and females in both the white and the black populations. In fact, when the downward trend was first observed, there was considerable debate about whether the decrease in coronary heart disease mortality was "real." Today there is little doubt that the death rate has declined and continues to do so. Moreover, the downward trend is occurring throughout several developed countries. The difficulties encountered in the search for the reasons underlying this significant downward trend are particularly interesting.

The major difficulty in this search stems from the number of factors believed to contribute to cardiovascular diseases generally and to coronary heart disease specifically. Ischemic heart disease has been referred to as a "malady of the civilized world." Increased risks for coronary heart disease include aging, increased cholesterol levels, obesity, sedentary or otherwise inactive lifestyles, smoking, and alcohol consumption, as well as numerous dietary and other lifestyle factors commonly associated with lifestyles in more developed countries. Hypertension and diabetes have also been designated as risk factors for coronary heart disease.

It remains unclear whether changing lifestyles, public health interventions with regard to early detection and prevention of coronary heart disease, or improved medical care for people afflicted with heart disease separately or in some combination are responsible for the observed decline. Some believe that campaigns by physicians and the public health sector geared toward cessation of smoking, altering diets, and increased exercise have had immediate results. However, it is questionable whether these changes have been widespread enough and have persisted for a time period sufficiently long to be strongly associated with the decline. Other evidence confuses the issue. For example, the number of women who smoke continues to increase among certain age segments, yet coronary heart disease declines. The search for an explanation continues. What we do know is that there has been and continues to be considerable variation in the geographic distribution of coronary or ischemic heart disease.

Geographic Patterns in Mortality Rates

1950. In 1950 heart diseases accounted for about 37 percent of all deaths. The 1950 age-adjusted death rates for coronary heart disease among white males and white females in the United States present an interesting and thought-provoking geographic pattern, as shown in Figures 5.1 and 5.2.

Among white males the death rate ranged from a low of 191 per 100,000 in New Mexico to 394 per 100,000 in New York. What is particularly notable is the major cluster of northeastern and New England states with especially high coronary disease death rates of at least 300 per 100,000. In addition to New York, other states in the very high death rate category included Rhode Island, Connecticut, New Hampshire, Delaware, New Jersey, Pennsylvania, and Maryland. In the West, California and Nevada were included in this category, and in the Deep South, Louisiana was included.

At the other extreme, low mortality rates of under 230 per 100,000 for white males were found in states of the South, such as Kentucky, Tennessee, Mississippi, and Alabama, as well as in the upper midwestern states of North Dakota and South Dakota.

Among white females the age-adjusted death rates from coronary heart disease in 1950 were much lower than those for white males. Rates ranged from a low of 83 per 100,000 in New Mexico to a high of 217 in New York, the same states with the lowest and highest mortality rates for white males. The geographic distribution of age-adjusted death rates among white females (Figure 5.2) closely mirrored that for white males. There was an even more pronounced concentration of very high death rates in the northeastern quadrant of the United States. States in a solid block from Maine to Pennsylvania and Maryland had mortality rates of at least 138 per 100,000. Only Illinois, Nevada, and California had death rates as high. In terms of geographic

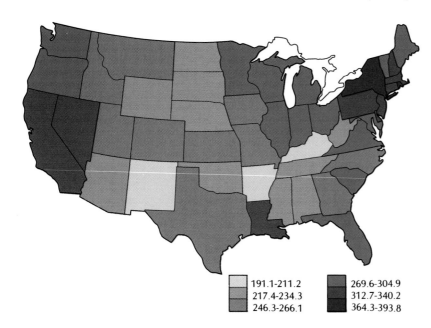

FIGURE 5.1

Coronary Heart Disease Mortality Rates for White Males (Deaths per 100,000 population), 1950

191.1-211.2   269.6-304.9
217.4-234.3   312.7-340.2
246.3-266.1   364.3-393.8

FIGURE 5.2

Coronary Heart Disease Mortality Rates for White Females (Deaths per 100,000 population), 1950

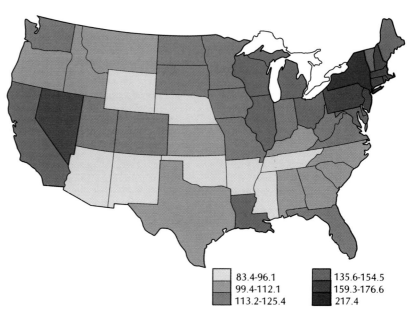

83.4-96.1   135.6-154.5
99.4-112.1   159.3-176.6
113.2-125.4 217.4

distribution, very low death rates of 100 per 100,000 and below for white females, like those for white males, were found in southern states such as Mississippi and Tennessee. Death rates of about 90 per 100,000 and below were found in Arkansas, Nebraska, Arizona, and Wyoming.

Thus, the geographic distributions of high and low coronary heart disease death rates for males and females were similar. Apparently, whatever the causes were, they affected white males and white females in about the same manner. Though it might be tempting to speculate that the patterns were associated with the relative urbanization of states, there was sufficient variation in urbanization in each category to negate this possible conclusion.

1968–1972. Age-adjusted coronary heart disease mortality data are available for the period 1968–1972 for black and white populations of the United States aged 35 to 74 (Figures 5.3 to 5.6). The geographic distributions of age-adjusted coronary heart disease mortality for white females and white males are illustrated in Figures 5.4 and 5.6.

Among white females, the average mortality rate was 217 per 100,000, and the mortality rate ranged from a low of 147 per 100,000 in Utah to a high of 275 per 100,000 in Delaware. Among white males, the average coronary heart disease mortality was 610 per 100,000; the rate ranged from a low of 428 per 100,000 in New Mexico to a very high 744 per 100,000 in South Carolina.

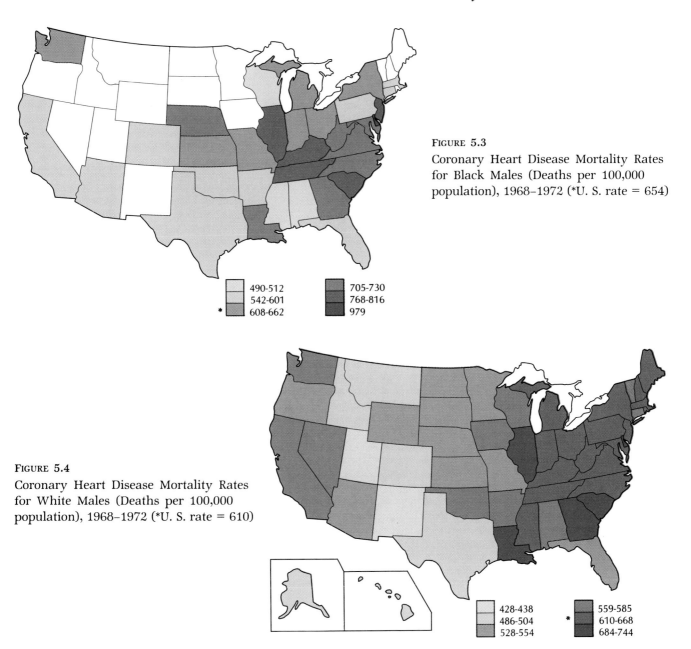

FIGURE 5.3

Coronary Heart Disease Mortality Rates for Black Males (Deaths per 100,000 population), 1968–1972 (*U. S. rate = 654)

490-512
542-601
* 608-662
705-730
768-816
979

FIGURE 5.4

Coronary Heart Disease Mortality Rates for White Males (Deaths per 100,000 population), 1968–1972 (*U. S. rate = 610)

428-438
486-504
528-554
* 559-585
610-668
684-744

What is particularly notable about the geographic distribution of coronary disease death rates for both white females and white males was the concentration of highest rates in the eastern one-third of the United States. The highest death rates for white males occurred in the Northeast and in states along the South Atlantic Coast from North Carolina (662 per 100,000) to Georgia (684 per 100,000) as well as in "outliers" such as Illinois (684 per 100,000) and Louisiana (705 per 100,000).

The coronary disease mortality pattern for white females was quite similar to that for males. There did appear to be an even greater concentration of high death rates in the Northeast, from Maine (with 255 white female deaths per 100,000) through Ohio (238 per 100,000) and Illinois (257 per 100,000). In the South, Louisiana (236 per 100,000) and South Carolina (240 per 100,000) had very high death rates for white females.

Age-adjusted mortality rates are available for 1968–1972 for states with significant numbers of black residents (more than 10,000). During this period the national average coronary heart disease mortality rate for black males ranged from a low (in Mississippi) of 490 deaths per 100,000 to a high (in Delaware) of 979 deaths per 100,000, and the national average was 654 deaths per 100,000 people, considerably higher than that for white males during the same time period. For black females the national average was 406 per 100,000, almost twice that for white females. Among

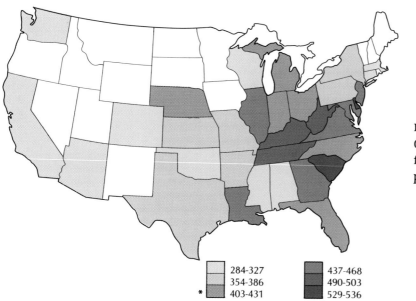

FIGURE 5.5
Coronary Heart Disease Mortality Rates for Black Females (Deaths per 100,000 population), 1968–1972 (*U. S. rate = 406)

FIGURE 5.6
Coronary Heart Disease Mortality Rates for White Females (Deaths per 100,000 population), 1968–1972 (*U. S. rate = 217)

the states considered here, the death rates ranged from a low of 284 per 100,000 in Washington to a high of 536 per 100,000 in South Carolina. Though the geographic data for black males and black females included only 17 states, the patterns appeared to be somewhat different from those for white males and white females. For example, with regard to black males for the period 1968–1972, the highest rates occurred in a cluster of states situated predominantly in the mid-South. This list included Kentucky (with 816 per 100,000), Tennessee (768 per 100,000), North Carolina and South Carolina (730 and 808 per 100,000, respectively), West Virginia and Virginia (727 and 725 per 100,000, respectively), and Maryland (714 per 100,000). Black males fared much better in the Deep

South, however, where some of the lowest coronary mortality rates occurred. Mississippi had a mortality rate of 490 per 100,000—the lowest among the states considered. Alabama (with 507 per 100,000) and Arkansas (542 per 100,000) also had very low rates relative to the other states included here.

A somewhat similar pattern occurred among black females (Figure 5.5). Again the mid-South states of South Carolina, Kentucky, West Virginia, Tennessee, and Virginia had among the highest coronary mortality rates, ranging from 536 per 100,000 population in South Carolina to 459 per 100,000 in Virginia. Outside this region, Delaware (with 529 per 100,000), Illinois (450 per 100,000), and New Jersey (440 per 100,000) also had very high mortality rates. With regard to the

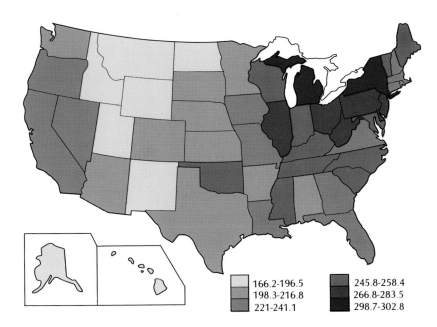

FIGURE 5.7

Coronary Heart Disease Mortality Rates, Total Population (Deaths per 100,000 Population), 1986

166.2-196.5   245.8-258.4
198.3-216.8   266.8-283.5
221-241.1   298.7-302.8

lowest rates, however, the black female pattern appeared to differ somewhat from the black male pattern. The lowest black female coronary mortality rates were found in Washington (284 per 100,000), Colorado (293 per 100,000), Oklahoma (304 per 100,000), and Wisconsin (308 per 100,000). The major difference in this pattern appeared to be the relatively less favorable positions of Mississippi, Alabama, and Arkansas for black females. These states had three of the four lowest mortality rates for black males but ranked ninth, tenth, and twelfth in mortality rates for black females. Generally, however, the geographic patterns for black males and black females were not very dissimilar, as was the case also for white males and white females.

1986. In 1986 the national average age-adjusted death rate from coronary heart disease was 246 per 100,000 people. As mentioned above, it accounted for almost 600,000 deaths, or 28 percent of all deaths during 1986. Death rates ranged from a low of 166 per 100,000 in Hawaii to 303 per 100,000 in New York. The geographic distribution of heart disease death rates for the total population by state is presented in Figure 5.7.

Particularly notable, as in the distributions for 1950 and 1968–1972, was the continuing concentration and further consolidation of highest death rates in the eastern third of the nation, especially in the northeastern quadrant. With the exception of Connecticut (which had a rate of 229 per 100,000), Massachusetts (239 per 100,000), Vermont (250 per 100,000), and New Hampshire (241 per 100,000), there was a solid tier of states from Maine (257 per 100,000) to New York (303 per 100,000) to Michigan (299 per 100,000) and Illinois (274 per 100,000) which had coronary heart disease rates higher than 250 per 100,000.

At the other end of the mortality spectrum, there was a contiguous north-to-south belt of ten states extending from a northern tier of states bounded by Minnesota and Idaho to the southern states of Arkansas, Texas, and New Mexico, which had among the lowest coronary heart disease mortality rates in the United States. Eight of these states had mortality rates of below 200 per 100,000 population. These included New Mexico (184 per 100,000), Utah (189 per 100,000), Idaho (190 per 100,000), North Dakota (192 per 100,000), Montana (195 per 100,000), Wyoming (197 per 100,000), Minnesota (198 per 100,000), and Arkansas (199 per 100,000). While the rates in this belt of states were much below the national average, the lowest rate occurred in Hawaii, one of the states most recently (1959) added to the United States, which had a rate of only 166 deaths per 100,000 people. This substantial difference may have been due to the racial mixture of the Hawaiian population, which is dominated by people of Asian descent. For example, people of Japanese origin constitute almost 25 percent of the population, and the Japanese historically have had the lowest coronary heart disease mortality rates among all developed countries, averaging about 100 deaths per 100,000 people annually. Alaska, the other state added in 1959, also has a very low mortality rate of 190 per 100,000 people.

Again, these strong state and regional coronary heart disease mortality differences add interest to the question of the unknown factors behind the declining rates in the United States. Do the populations with high rates continue to practice poor health habits and thus have higher death rates? Or is the care of the heart attack victim in these areas such that survival rates are not as high as in other states? The answers to these questions are that we do not know which factor

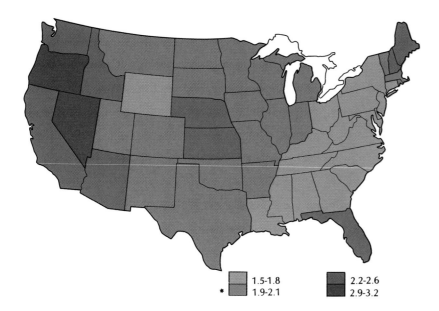

FIGURE 5.8
Ischemic Heart Disease Mortality, Male-to-Female Ratio, 1940 (*U. S. average = 1.9)

FIGURE 5.9
Ischemic Heart Disease Mortality, Male-to-Female Ratio, 1960 (*U. S. average = 3.5)

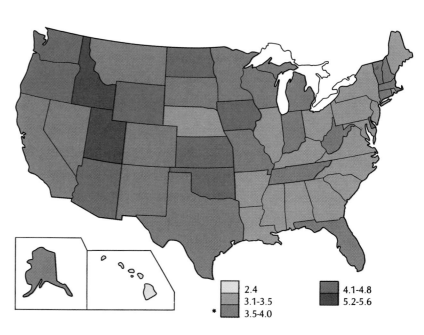

or combination of factors is responsible. Further confounding the search for underlying causal factors is a parallel decline in coronary heart disease mortality in several other developed countries, beginning also in the mid to late 1960s. Is there perhaps some common yet unknown factor involved? The search continues, and the coronary heart disease mortality rate continues to decline, even while coronary heart disease remains the major killer disease in the United States.

Male-to-Female Mortality Ratios

One curiosity pertaining to coronary heart disease is the consistently and significantly higher mortality

the geographic distribution of male-to-female mortality ratios. In other words, though females have consistently lower mortality rates than males, we are interested in examining the ratio of male mortality to female mortality for each state. These national patterns are presented in Figures 5.8 to 5.16.

1940. In 1940, according to statistics compiled on coronary heart disease mortality, nationally almost two males died for every female who died (Figure 5.8). However, the ratios ranged from a low of 1.5:1 to a high of 3.2:1. The highest ratios, with coronary death rates for men over 3 times as high as those for women, occurred in Oregon and Nevada. These states are contiguous to other western states, including Washington, California, Idaho, and Arizona, where, in 1940 at least,

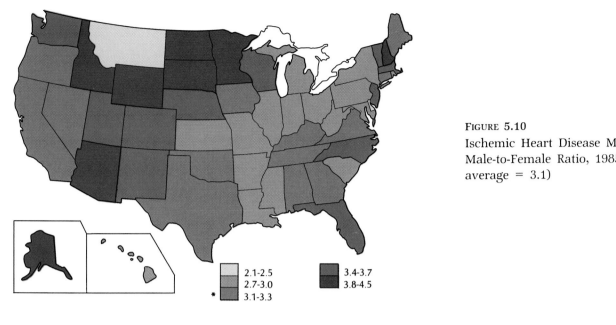

FIGURE 5.10
Ischemic Heart Disease Mortality, Male-to-Female Ratio, 1985 (*U. S. average = 3.1)

2.1-2.5	3.4-3.7
2.7-3.0	3.8-4.5
* 3.1-3.3	

FIGURE 5.11
Ischemic Heart Disease, Premature Male Mortality, 1940 (*U. S. average = 397)

218-280	420-457
294-348	464-509
* 364-410	

men were dying from coronary heart disease at rates over twice as high as those of females. Similar differentials were found in Nebraska and Kansas in the Midwest, Maine and New Hampshire in the far Northeast, and Florida in the extreme Southeast.

1960. The national average ratio of male deaths to female deaths from coronary heart disease increased to 3.5:1 by 1960 (Figure 5.9). This means that, on average, almost four men died from coronary heart disease for each female death. In contrast to 1940, every state had over two males dying for each female death by 1960. As in 1940, states with the lowest ratios in 1960, in this case 2.4:1 to 3.0:1, were distributed primarily in the eastern third of the nation. The higher ratios are found in western states.

rates among men. This pattern occurs not only in the United States but throughout the developed countries for which mortality data are available. This difference persists in countries with the highest and lowest coronary heart disease mortality rates. In Finland, for example, over a recent 20-year period, the mortality rate for males aged 35 to 74 averaged about 900 deaths per 100,000 persons. For females in the same age category, however, the death rate was less than 300 per 100,000, or about one-third the male death rate. In Japan the average annual mortality rate was just over 100 per 100,000 for males and approximately 50 per 100,000 for females—about half the rate for males.

We have shown that the geographic distribution of coronary heart disease mortality rates for females and males is similar. It is interesting, however, to examine

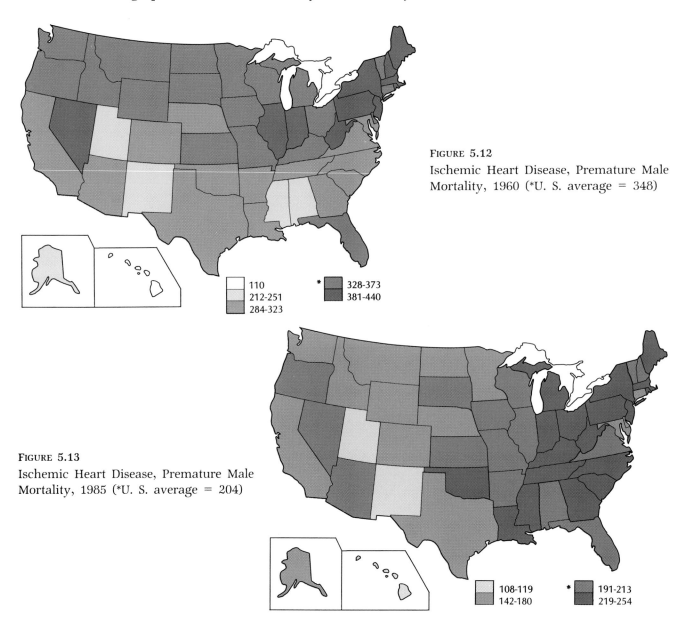

FIGURE 5.12
Ischemic Heart Disease, Premature Male
Mortality, 1960 (*U. S. average = 348)

	110	*	328-373
	212-251		381-440
	284-323		

FIGURE 5.13
Ischemic Heart Disease, Premature Male
Mortality, 1985 (*U. S. average = 204)

	108-119	*	191-213
	142-180		219-254

Rather amazingly high male-to-female ratios of coronary heart disease mortality, 5.2:1 and 5.6:1, were found in Idaho and Utah. In these states, for each female who died of coronary heart disease, more than five males died of the same problem. High male-to-female ratios, ranging from 4.1:1 to 4.8:1, were found again in such states as Washington and Arizona. A notable change took place in Nebraska relative to the rest of the country between 1940 and 1960. In 1940 Nebraska had a relatively very high male-to-female ratio (2.3:1); in 1960 the ratio was 2.4:1. Thus, though Nebraska's ratio remained stable between 1940 and 1960, yet by 1960 it had become one of the lowest ratios in the country.

1985. By 1985, the national average male-to-female ratio of coronary heart disease mortality had declined to 3.1:1.0 (Figure 5.10). Still, approximately three males were dying from coronary heart disease for each female death. The highest ratios, from 3.8:1 to 4.5:1, were found in a northern tier of states extending from Minnesota to Idaho. There was also a reemergence of high rates in the East, from New Hampshire, Vermont, and Massachusetts in the Northeast southward through New Jersey to North Carolina and Florida. Very high rates continued in states such as Utah and Arizona, as well as in New Mexico and Colorado.

In 1985 the differential between male and female rates of coronary heart disease remained a consistent feature in the health and death experience of the United States. Without exception, in the years included in this chapter, the male death rate exceeded the female. However, historically as well as currently there has been considerable geographic variation in male

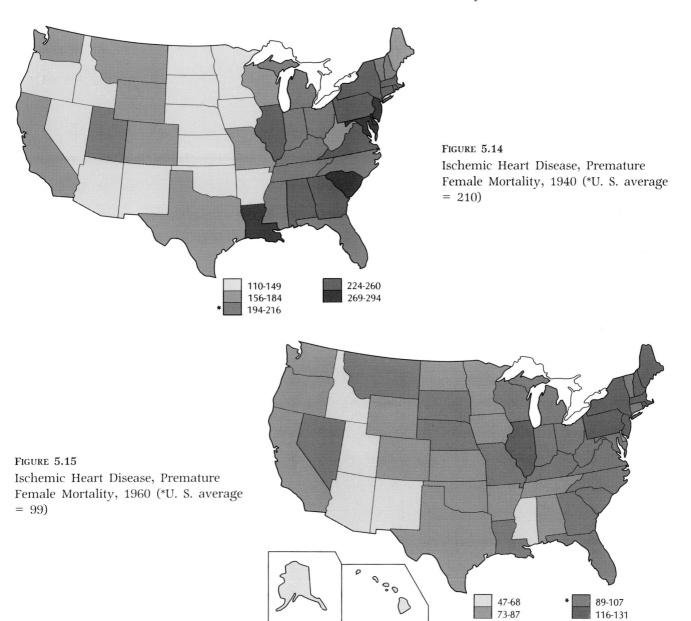

FIGURE 5.14
Ischemic Heart Disease, Premature Female Mortality, 1940 (*U. S. average = 210)

110-149		224-260	
156-184		269-294	
* 194-216			

FIGURE 5.15
Ischemic Heart Disease, Premature Female Mortality, 1960 (*U. S. average = 99)

47-68		* 89-107	
73-87		116-131	

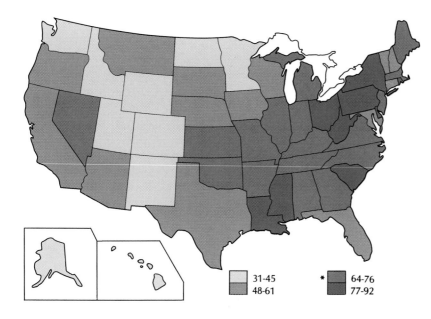

FIGURE 5.16
Ischemic Heart Disease, Premature Female Mortality, 1985 (*U. S. average = 66)

31-45
48-61
* 64-76
77-92

and female mortality rates. In some states "only" two males die from coronary heart disease for each female who dies. In other states, however, for each female who dies, almost five males die. The underlying reasons for this substantial differential remain elusive. The observed geographic differences may be due to local differences in diet, smoking patterns, obesity, and a host of other factors that have been implicated in coronary heart disease. Again, the number and complexity of purported underlying factors makes finding an explanation for the wide range of male-to-female mortality ratios difficult.

6

Cerebrovascular Disease

Cerebrovascular disease (also known as "stroke") can be manifested by the abrupt onset of multiple conditions. Loss of speech and/or the use of all or some of the arms and legs often takes place. A very mild stroke may result in only short-term disability, but a very severe stroke can lead to permanent disability or possibly even death. A stroke can begin with loss of consciousness, but early symptoms often include only blurred vision and dizziness. Strokes often happen between midnight and 6:00 A.M., when the human body is functioning at minimal levels. Frequently, either the right or the left side of the body is affected, depending upon which half of the brain suffers damage.

A stroke results from a disturbed blood supply that leads to an inadequate flow to the brain. The disruption may be due to several different conditions. Two of these conditions are classified as "ischemia" or "infarction"—(see the section on coronary heart disease) and "hemorrhage." The vascular disorders that are considered ischemic are cerebral thrombosis and cerebral embolism. Cerebral thrombosis occurs when the blood supply to the brain is restricted due to atherosclerosis. Deposits of fatty tissue can break free from artery walls and contribute to blood clots that lead to blockage. Cerebral embolism is also a form of blockage, in this instance created by some kind of extraneous material that blocks an artery. About three-quarters of all strokes are due to infarction.

The other one-quarter of cases of cerebrovascular disease are due to hemorrhage. This circumstance is usually brought about by either a form of arterial hypertension or a ruptured artery that leaks. Blood is diverted from arteries and clots form. A hemorrhage can be more serious than either form of thrombosis. There is therefore a higher probability of death resulting from a hemorrhage.

During most of this century, cerebrovascular disease has been a leading cause of death. Since the 1940s it has ranked third highest, behind heart disease and cancer. Although cerebral hemorrhage especially can happen at any age, most stroke victims are 65 years of age or older. Elderly persons are generally at higher risk because they have more atherosclerosis and usually higher blood pressure than younger persons. Since both of these conditions increase with age, frequent blood pressure checks and dietary control are the best preventive measures against stroke. While preventive behavior in general lowers the probability of stroke, often the condition cannot be prevented. About one-third of strokes are fatal, particularly for persons over 80 years old. Another third can lead to some form of disability, and yet another third result in no permanent impairments.

Early Reporting Systems in the United States

The systematic reporting of information about cerebrovascular disease in the United States dates mostly to the beginning of this century. Two states, Massachusetts and New Jersey, started collecting and publishing such information in the 1880s. Most of the remainder of New England as well as New York State started for-

55

mal reporting by 1890. By 1910, more than 20 states were regularly reporting information about death due to cerebrovascular disease to the U.S. Public Health Service, and only a dozen remained as nonreporting states by 1920. During the early 1930s a regular nationwide reporting system for cerebrovascular disease deaths was intact.

Reporting by racial category started by 1910 but also was not comprehensive until the 1930s. In addition, during the 1930s categories such as "white" and "nonwhite" varied considerably, with Mexicans and Puerto Ricans sometimes considered white and sometimes nonwhite before 1940. Likewise, the nonwhite categories sometimes included blacks, native Americans, and Asians.

Given such data reporting limitations, it is still important to understand longer-term trends in stroke mortality. For example, for the year 1900 the age-adjusted death rate for cerebrovascular disease for all races and both sexes was 134.4 deaths per 100,000 population. During that year there were only minor differences between male (136.9 per 100,000) and female (132.2 per 100,000) rates. As mentioned, no racial breakdowns are available for the first two decades of this century. By 1920, the overall age-adjusted death rate for cerebrovascular disease was 122.6 deaths per 100,000 persons, with more significant differences between the male (118.2 per 100,000) and female (127.2 per 100,000) rates. The overall rate for white persons in 1920 was 120.8 per 100,000 (117.3 for men and 124.2 for women). Conversely, the mortality rate from cerebrovascular disease for black persons was 145.8 per 100,000, which was higher than the overall national rate in 1900. In addition, there were substantial differences between nonwhite females and nonwhite males in 1920. Nonwhite females had a rate of 170.6 per 100,000 and nonwhite males had a rate of 125.2 per 100,000, which was somewhat close to the overall national average.

Reports of age breakdowns during the period 1900–1940 also offer some useful historical background information for this disease. During this time period, all age groups below 55 years old had mortality rates lower than the national average for any given year. Rates increased with age. The 55-to-64-year-old group, for example, reported rates twice as high as the national average. Still, in 1900, the death rate for the 55-to-64-year-old group was 319.6 per 100,000 population; by 1920, it was 286.9, and by 1940, it was 211.8. By contrast, rates also more than doubled for the 65-to-70-year-old group during the early decades of this century. Thus, by 1900 the rate per 100,000 for people between 65 and 74 years of age was 828.2; by 1920, it was 809.1, and by 1940, it was 573.8. The rates for people over 75 years of age for all years during the

first part of this century was also more than double the rate for the younger age cohort. More precisely, at the beginning of World War II, the mortality rate from cerebrovascular disease for persons born on the eve of the Civil War was approximately 2,500 per 100,000.

Geographic Patterns in Mortality Rates

1940. The geographic distribution of stroke deaths in 1940 was as striking as were the differences by age groups. The pattern shown in Figure 6.1 is an excellent example of the extreme geographical clustering of this chronic and degenerative disease. For example, rates for 1940 were above the national average of 91 per 100,000 population west of the Mississippi River and considerably below the average in the western United States. The heaviest concentrations of much higher than average rates were in the South Atlantic states. The clustering of highest incidence states during that period included Virginia, North Carolina, South Carolina, Georgia, and Florida. All the high-incidence states in 1940 were located east of the Mississippi River. A group of midwestern states, as well as some states in the South Central parts of the country, reported 1940 rates somewhat above average. West Virginia, Maryland, Delaware, Vermont, and Maine also had above-average rates. With the exception of New York State, the states with the lowest incidence of stroke mortality in 1940 were located in the more youthful, southwestern parts of the United States, including Utah, Colorado, Arizona, New Mexico, Nevada, and California. The entire central tier of states in the United States from the Dakotas and Minnesota in the North through the Great Plains to Oklahoma and Texas in the South, as well as the Pacific Northwest states, were all below the national average in 1940. This general east-west contrast in stroke mortality has remained consistent throughout the twentieth century.

Some but not all of the 1940 east-west differences can be attributed to differential stroke rates in white and nonwhite categories. In 1940 the overall white stroke mortality rate was 85.7 per 100,000, with rates of 87.9 for males and 83.4 for females. A significant difference was reported for nonwhite persons. The overall nonwhite rate was 151.8 per 100,000, with 141.8 for males and 162.6 for females. Note that the stroke mortality rate for nonwhite females was almost double that for white females.

1960. By the early 1960s, approximately 200,000 deaths attributed to cerebrovascular disease were reported annually. These deaths accounted for about 12 percent of deaths from all causes in the United States and for about 20 percent of all deaths among people under 65 years of age. The marked east-west geographical contrast in stroke deaths continued. The pattern shown in Figure 6.2 for 1960 demonstrates this trend. While there was still higher than average stroke mortality in the southeastern parts of the United States, somewhat higher than average rates were also reported for many states east of the Mississippi River. Unlike the 1940s pattern, several states west of the Mississippi (Texas, Oklahoma, and Oregon) reported rates above the national average of 86 deaths per 100,000 persons in 1960. Generally, states in the western part of the United States were average or below for stroke deaths by 1960. In addition, a cluster of states in the northeastern United States (New York, New Jersey, Pennsylvania, Maryland, and Delaware) continued to report stroke death rates below the national average.

Overall, stroke mortality rates showed an increase in many parts of the United States from 1940 to 1950; however, there was a clear drop in rates for almost all states from 1950 to 1960. For both white and nonwhite population groups, the risk of stroke continued to increase with age. By 1960 also, the risk was generally higher for males than for females, particularly in the more elderly groups. Examination of some representative states for the period 1940–1960 helps to explain both male-female and white-nonwhite differences in stroke death rates. For example, Michigan, a state at about the national average in 1960, had actually reported higher stroke death rates for both males and females in 1950 than in 1940. By 1960, however, Michigan was reporting much lower rates. The 1960 white male stroke mortality rate in Michigan was 86.1 per 100,000 population, a rate near the national average, just as it had been in 1940. The nonwhite stroke mortality in Michigan in 1960 was 121.9 per 100,000, with 112.9 for males and 130.9 for females.

This gender difference was not consistent from one state to another. In other words, not all states reported higher nonwhite female than nonwhite male mortality for 1960.

One of the highest rates for 1960 was reported by Georgia. The overall Georgia rate was 136.8 per 100,000 population, with a male rate of 146.4 and a female rate of 129.3. The rate was 115.3 for white males, and the rate for white females was 92.3. In sharp contrast, the nonwhite stroke mortality rate (236.8 per 100,000) was almost double the white rate. The state's black male rate was 243.1 per 100,000, and the black female rate was 232.3 per 100,000—more than double the white female rate.

Stroke mortality in Colorado in 1960 exemplifies a state at the other end of the spectrum. The overall Colorado rate was 73.4 per 100,000 population, with 69.1 for males and 77.1 for females. Few differences were reported between white and nonwhite groups in Colorado, a state with a very small minority population at that time.

One of the most noteworthy features of the decades immediately prior to World War II was a general downward trend in overall cerebrovascular disease mortality. This trend showed up particularly among middle-aged white persons in the United States. Part of this circumstance can be attributed to general improvements in health care conditions in the country during the post-World War II period. In addition, it can be assumed that as physician's understanding of arterial hypertension increased, so did their abilities to treat patients. Yet another reason for the declining rates included public education programs and the earlier detection of some of the conditions that might lead to stroke. A haunting impression of regional variations in stroke mortality still persisted in the 1960s, however. It became increasingly clear, as reporting for white and nonwhite groups improved, that there were markedly higher stroke mortality rates for black persons, both male and female. In addition, the southeastern states with the highest concentrations of black people continued to show the highest concentrations of stroke death reporting. Many county-based studies of stroke mortality since the 1950s have corroborated this conclusion.

The 1970s and the Early 1980s. In the late 1970s and the early 1980s, downward trends in stroke mortality rates continued to be clearly apparent in the United States as well as in many other parts of the world. Public health workers have determined that this downward trend actually began to accelerate during the early 1970s. During most of the 1970s and the first half of the 1980s, the chances of mortality by stroke for most age groups dropped considerably, at least for individuals under 75 years old. Among nonwhite persons there was an even greater rate of decline for all persons under 65 years of age. This statistic, of course, has much to do with the fact that overall rates during earlier parts of the century were much higher for nonwhite persons than for people classified as white. By the mid-1980s, chances of stroke mortality were consistently higher for men, regardless of race, than for women. Overall, during most of the 1970s and 1980s, stroke mortality rates for most age groups dropped as much as 1 percent per year. The heaviest geographical concentrations of stroke mortality in the United States continued to occur in the southeastern part of the country during the 1970s. High stroke death rates per 100,000 population for white males between 35 and 74 years of age were most heavily concentrated in Mississippi and Alabama; in parts of the coal mining regions of Appalachia; and in the coastal plains of North Caro-

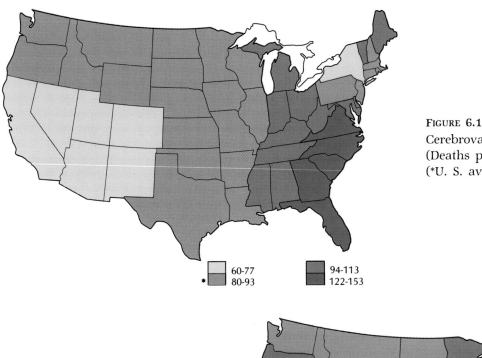

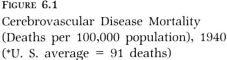

FIGURE 6.1
Cerebrovascular Disease Mortality
(Deaths per 100,000 population), 1940
(*U. S. average = 91 deaths)

	60-77		94-113
*	80-93		122-153

FIGURE 6.2
Cerebrovascular Disease Mortality
(Deaths per 100,000 population), 1960
(*U. S. average = 86 deaths)

	61-74		87-102
*	76-86		110-137

lina, South Carolina, and Georgia. This regional concentration persisted during the 1980s. Stroke mortality patterns for white females aged 35 to 74 during the 1970s and the 1980s were somewhat more widespread, but there were still some concentrations of higher incidence in the Coastal Plains areas of the southeastern U.S. It has become increasingly clear that parts of the United States can now be more easily identified as *endemic* areas for higher probabilities of stroke mortality in both men and women. In fact, the relationship is essentially one of higher stroke mortality for both men and women in poorer regions of the United States (i.e. the Southeast), with lower overall rates occurring in more prosperous areas of the country.

The trends discussed above, which have been clearly identified within the United States, are similar to differences in stroke mortality on an international level,

between more developed and less developed countries. Even so, examination of more developed industrialized nations also shows a range of different stroke mortality rates. For example, Norway, Sweden, and Denmark reported some of the lowest stroke mortality rates in the world during the 1980s. Low stroke rates also characterized the populations of The Netherlands, Switzerland, and Canada. Developed countries with somewhat higher rates included Czechoslovakia, Austria, and Japan. However, recent studies have shown that stroke mortality rates in Japan are also on the decrease. Developed countries with stroke mortality rates in the intermediate range include the United States and the United Kingdom.

Some differences by gender have also become apparent, particularly during the 1980s. For example, in France, Austria, and Switzerland females experienced

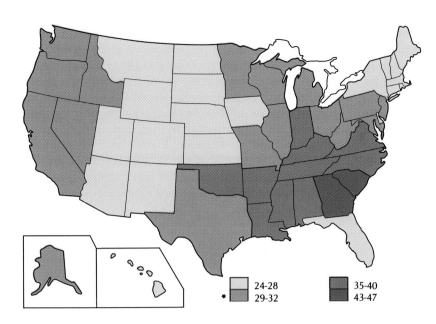

FIGURE 6.3
Cerebrovascular Disease Mortality
(Deaths per 100,000 population),
1985–1987 (*U. S. average = 31 deaths)

24-28	35-40
29-32	43-47

a much stronger decline in stroke mortality rates than did males. Japan, which had a higher stroke mortality during the 1960s and 1970s, has in more recent decades experienced a decline of up to 7 percent per year among both males and females. As information has become increasingly available for Eastern European countries, evidence has been developing which indicates that stroke mortality rates have not declined much in the past couple of decades. In some countries—Hungary, Poland, and Bulgaria, for example—stroke mortality rates in men actually increased during the 1970s and the 1980s. Countries that have shown little change in stroke mortality rates since the 1970s include Yugoslavia, Romania, and Czechoslovakia. During the late 1980s, several developed countries, including the United States and Australia, experienced declines in stroke mortality rates of about 5 percent per year among both men and women.

Several factors appear to be contributing to either a lack of decline or, in some instances, to real increases in stroke mortality rates in some developing countries. Problems with environmental contamination in Eastern Europe are now well documented. While these conditions may not contribute directly to stroke mortality, conditions such as hypertension have a higher probability of developing. The link between stroke and hypertension has been demonstrated. It is expected that stroke mortality rates in Eastern Europe will decline during the remainder of the 1990s, as economic conditions improve, yielding better health conditions.

The Late 1980s. Many of the complex factors that result in higher stroke mortality internationally are also apparently operating in the United States. The familiar pattern of southeastern U.S. concentrations of excessive stroke deaths, which had been identified in earlier pe-

riods, persisted during the late 1980s (Figure 6.3). Two states, South Carolina and Georgia, reported the highest stroke mortality rates in the United States during the period 1985–1987. In addition, the Coastal Plains continued to report higher-than-average mortality rates. States reporting higher-than-average incidence were North Carolina, Virginia, Kentucky, Tennessee, Georgia, Alabama, Louisiana, and Arkansas. Oklahoma and Indiana reported higher-than-average rates during the same period. Most of the remainder of the United States had rates below the national average of 31 deaths per 100,000 persons. The lowest rates in the United States during the late 1980s occurred in New England, Florida, and the central tier of states in the western United States. The West Coast continued to report stroke mortality rates far below the national average. In spite of an overall decline in stroke mortality, southeastern parts of the country maintained their traditional high rates.

Conclusion

Declines in overall cerebrovascular disease mortality continue to be the subject of geographical research because of the regional clustering of stroke cases. Extensive studies of hypertension have been conducted in the southeastern Coastal Plains areas of the United States. Studies of interest include the monitoring of the blood pressure of high school students in selected cities, such as Savannah, Georgia. To date, the indications are that socioeconomic factors outweigh any predisposition to stroke mortality on the basis of inherited factors that might be specifically linked to race.

Several explanations of the overall decreases in stroke mortality have been offered. It has been suggested that earlier detection of individual propensity toward stroke has enabled physicians to treat potential victims with certain kinds of preventive measures, including diet and medication. Tremendous progress has been made in the reduction of stroke mortality among several age groups during the last couple of decades. Overall declines in stroke mortality have been achieved among the 55-to-64-year-old group, the 65-to-70-year-old group, and even the 75-to-84-year-old group. There are less accurate data for people aged 85 and older. During the past 20 years, perhaps as many as 0.25 million people have been spared death from cerebrovascular disease in the United States—a number of people equivalent to the population of a medium-sized metropolitan area. In addition, perhaps as many as 0.50 million more lives have been saved after nonfatal strokes. As progress in combating stroke mortality continues, geographical concentrations remain the same. Such important aspects of lifestyle change as stopping cigarette smoking, making changes in diet, cutting back on use of alcohol, and participating in exercise programs have contributed to decreased stroke mortality. The greatest challenge for the remainder of this century appears to be combating differential stroke mortality due to economic conditions.

7

Cancer

From 15 to 16 percent of all deaths in the United States during the late twentieth century will be attributed to some form of cancer. Cancer is second only to heart disease as a leading cause of death. Just as there are many forms of heart disease, there are also different kinds of cancer. However, though the various diseases of the circulatory system affect somewhat limited parts of the human body, the different forms of cancer can affect a wide variety of areas of the human body. In fact, the many forms of cancer are referred to by some researchers as different diseases.

Cancer has been defined as uncontrolled new growth which invades and destroys living tissue. Cancerous growths are made up of cells that differ from normal cells in size, shape, and growth rates, among other ways. Malignant tumors (carcinomas), the first of the two major types of cancer, are, of course, different from benign ones and are characterized by growth beyond the body organ of origin. In general, malignant tumors demonstrate a higher rate of cell growth and multiplication than normal tissues. The growth is uncontrolled, and thus there is a complete lack of tissue and organ boundary maintenance. Malignant tumors also have a microscopic appearance which suggests immature rather than mature cells. The other major form of cancer is sarcoma (soft-tissue cancer), or cancer that originates in connective tissue or bone. Because of these histological implications, cancers have traditionally been considered a collection of diseases rather than a single type of disease. In addition, there are different cancer rates by location in the body that have been attributed to differences in sex, age, race, place of residence, individual behavior, environment, and specific "insults" or injuries to the body.

Historically shrouded in mystery, for centuries cancer has been known as an occasionally rapid and sometimes unexpected cause of death. The lives of many central figures in history have been ended by cancer. Ancient Egyptians knew of both major forms of cancer, tumors and sarcomas. Because of the crablike shape of some forms of cancer, the ancient Greeks referred to the disease as *karkinoma*. Western culture inherited the Latin word for "crab," *cancer*, from the Romans. The Egyptians, the Greeks, and the Romans all practiced various forms of surgery in attempts to remove tumors, and there is evidence that many early cultures were aware of the importance of removing some tumors as soon as possible. Various accounts of cancer during the Middle Ages can be found.

As the Industrial Revolution brought about rapid growth of cities in Europe during the late 1700s, some scholars drew associations between industrialization and certain forms of cancer. At about the same time, there were reports of lung cancer problems among European coal miners. By the 1800s, cancer had taken on a clear association with modernization in various cultures. Two major theories about the causes of cancer were popular by the end of the nineteenth century. One of these theories held that cancer was contagious. To some extent this kind of thinking was inadvertently exacerbated by the microbiological discoveries of Robert Koch, Louis Pasteur, and others during the late nineteenth century, which led some people to think that cancer was spread by "germs." The second major

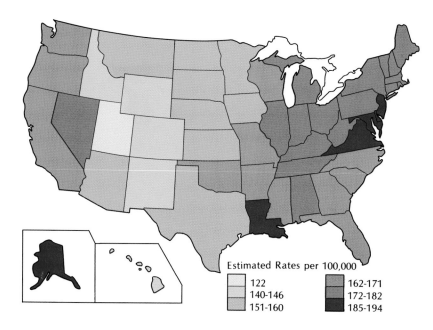

FIGURE 7.1
Cancer Death Rates for All Sites in 1990

Estimated Rates per 100,000

122	162-171
140-146	172-182
151-160	185-194

theory was that certain people carried cancerous genes. The idea that cancer could be genetic was offered some support by investigators who found small but very important geographical clusters of certain kinds of the disease in specific villages and other locales.

It is now known that specific kinds of behavior—for example, the use of tobacco products and/or alcohol abuse—can lead to cancer. In addition, there is extensive proof that heart disease, lung cancer, and emphysema are all directly linked to tobacco consumption. At the beginning of the twentieth century, most smokers were addicted to pipes and cigars, and society had not yet made an association between smoking and lung problems. There was, however, a general awareness that cancers of the mouth and throat could develop as a result of extensive smoking. Throughout the early part of the twentieth century, the major treatment for cancer was surgery. The disease had certain "sinister" aspects; many people were unwilling to discuss cancer. Part of the cancer denial ethic can be attributed to lack of understanding of the causes of cancer. A social stigma had developed, coupled with persistent fears of contagion. Increasingly, during the early part of the twentieth century, incipient epidemiological studies placed emphasis on behavioral aspects of cancer risks. Some early researchers hypothesized that there were dietary causes of some forms of cancer. It was suggested that cultures in which there was high consumption of such foods as pasta and rice generally had lower cancer rates than those in which there was high meat consumption. Other possible indicators that started to emerge included stress and a general increase in cancer risk with increasing age.

As society progressed into the modern medical era, and as the discovery of viruses in the 1930s led to further development of vaccines during the 1940s, some researchers also sought to discover a viral connection with cancer. Such an association, however, was not to be easily determined.

Although radium had been used as a treatment for cancer during the early part of this century, the increased use of chemotherapy by the 1950s and 1960s was in keeping with increased medical knowledge. Improved cancer treatment also resulted from the rise of institutes for research in cancer. As early as the 1930s, the U.S. government established the National Cancer Institute as part of the National Institutes of Health. In addition, the American Cancer Society evolved during the mid-twentieth century. It became clear by the 1960s that combinations of treatment, including surgery, chemotherapy, and radiation, could be of tremendous assistance when some forms of cancer were caught during early stages.

Public information campaigns regarding the connection between cancer and tobacco consumption became increasingly widespread by the mid-1960s. Additional knowledge of other sources of cancer was provided to the general public, and by the 1970s, people in general had become more willing to discuss cancer as a leading cause of death. Besides tobacco, other carcinogens were identified, including asbestos, X rays, certain kinds of food additives, radiation, and in some instances particles in the air that people were breathing and substances in the water they were drinking. Cancer cases associated with the contaminated Love Canal stood out as an example of environmental outrage. In addition, during the 1970s the "cancer alley" that had developed in the urbanized northeastern corridor of the United States had been clearly identified as a cancer cluster region.

In the early 1990s cancer continues to be the second leading cause of death in the United States. In any given year during the late 1980s and the early 1990s, the crude death rate for all forms of cancer in the United States has been about 140 per 100,000 persons. This statistic translates into about 15 percent of all deaths in the United States during any given recent year. The geographical distribution of cancer death rates for all sites in 1990 is depicted in Figure 7.1. The most striking feature of this pattern is that the highest-incidence states are in the eastern part of the country. The Eastern Seaboard high-cancer incidence region clearly stands out, as Virginia, Maryland, Washington, D.C., Delaware, and New Jersey continue to report some of the highest cancer death rates in the United States. The entire northeastern manufacturing belt of the United States continues to report higher-than-

average cancer death rates. Another group of high-incidence states extends southward to include Kentucky, Tennessee, and Alabama. There is also a district cluster in the Mississippi Delta, with very high rates reported for Louisiana as well as some surrounding states. Yet another somewhat higher than average regional cluster is situated along the West Coast of the United States, in Washington, Oregon, and California. The Great Plains and Rocky Mountains areas of the United States generally report cancer death rates lower than the national average. None of these regional patterns is new. A detailed examination of specific forms of cancer mortality for earlier time periods assists in explaining some of the similarities and differences that have been reported in cancer death rates over time within the United States.

LUNG CANCER

Lung cancer is a major cause of death in the United States among both females and males. While the disease is much more widespread among males, lung cancer death rates have also been on the increase among females in recent years. However, the 1990 death rate from lung cancer among men was more than 2.5 times higher than that among women. Long-term trends are even more striking. In 1930, for example, the age-adjusted death rate for lung cancer among men averaged about 3 per 100,000, while the female rate was about 1.75 per 100,000 (Figures 7.2 and 7.3). During the period 1983–1987, the average age-adjusted rates were 26.3 for females and 73.9 for males. Obviously, the rate of increase for males has been phenomenal. Even after the Surgeon General's report explaining cancer risks associated with smoking was issued in 1964, the rate of lung cancer mortality among males continued to accelerate at a very rapid rate. However, a cross-sectional geographical analysis of lung cancer during two different time periods shows some shifting in the distribution of regional clusters.

Geographic Patterns in Mortality Rates

1930–1932. During the period 1930–1932, the average age-adjusted mortality rate for lung cancer among both females and males in the United States was only a fraction of what it is today. There were several pronounced regional clusters of both higher and lower lung cancer incidences. The pattern shown in Figure 7.4 is one of definite regional contrasts. The most sig-

nificant cluster of high incidence lung cancer during the 1930–1932 period included New York, New Jersey, Maryland, Massachusetts, and Connecticut. This Northeastern Seaboard cluster is of particular interest because it appears that the heavy geographical concentrations of lung cancer that were reported in the 1970s were already in formative stages by the 1930s. Another higher-than-average incidence area was located in the southwestern United States. This concentration is more difficult to explain, because in the 1930s there was little industry in this area. The southeastern United States was characterized by a much lower than average lung cancer incidence rate in the 1930s.

Only slight variations show up when the early 1930s data are examined separately for males and females. The high concentrations of lung cancer in both the Northeast and the Southwest show up when male lung cancer patterns are examined (Figure 7.2). In addition, the Southeast reported lower-than-average rates. Even when male data are separated from female data, the pattern appears to be similar. The female lung cancer distribution map for the period 1930–1932 (Figure 7.3) departs somewhat from the male pattern in subtle ways. While concentrations of higher-than-average lung cancer in the Northeast included both male and female rates, concentrations of higher-than-average rates in the Southwest were not so strong for females as for males. This aspect of regional distribution and clustering was somewhat contrasted with higher-than-average rates of female lung cancer in the upper Midwest. These 1930s distributional patterns of lung cancer may have set the stage for early regional clusters of higher and lower rates, but a more dispersed pattern showed up by the 1980s.

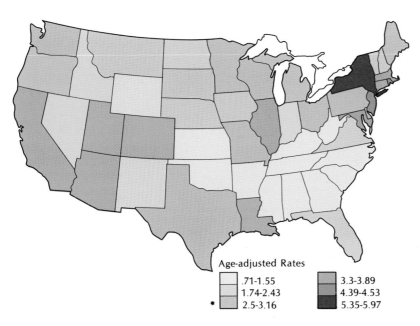

FIGURE 7.2

Male Lung Cancer Mortality Rates, 1930–1932 (*U. S. average = 3.01)

Age-adjusted Rates

.71-1.55   3.3-3.89
1.74-2.43   4.39-4.53
* 2.5-3.16   5.35-5.97

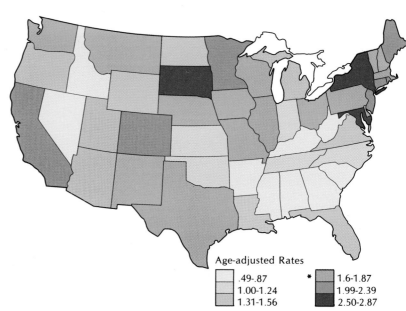

FIGURE 7.3

Female Lung Cancer Mortality Rates, 1930–1932 (*U. S. average = 1.74)

Age-adjusted Rates

.49-.87   * 1.6-1.87
1.00-1.24   1.99-2.39
1.31-1.56   2.50-2.87

The 1980s. Some geographical patterns of lung cancer mortality were the same in the 1980s as in the 1930s, but there were also some major changes. The information in Figure 7.5 helps to provide an understanding of the strong regional contrasts in lung cancer deaths for both males and females that had developed by the period 1983–1987. During that time the age-adjusted U.S. average was 46.4 deaths per 100,000 persons—15 times higher than the rate for the 1930–1932 period for the entire U.S. population. This distribution is unlike previous distributions in that the heaviest concentrations of much higher than average age-adjusted lung cancer death rates were in the southeastern United States. Core states for this region during the late 1980s were Kentucky, West Virginia, and Louisiana, with

much higher than average rates also in many adjacent states. In the western part of the United States, Nevada reported somewhat higher than average figures, along with California, Oregon, and Washington. As with total cancer death rates, the parts of the United States with the lowest incidence were in the Great Plains and Rocky Mountains regions. When female lung cancer mortality rates are separated from the total population, the highest-incidence region is definitely in the western United States. Nevada reported the highest overall female lung cancer mortality rates for the period 1983–1987, and much higher than average rates were reported for California, Oregon, and Washington (see Figure 7.6). Another somewhat higher than average cluster of female lung cancer mortality rates during the

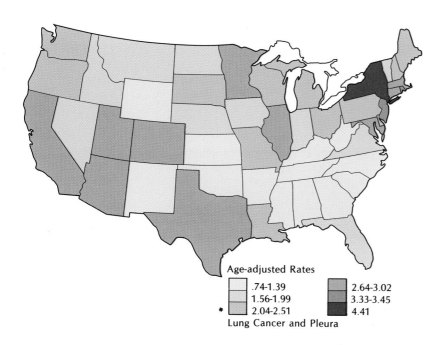

FIGURE 7.4

Male and Female Lung Cancer Mortality Rates, 1930–1932 (*U. S. average = 2.39)

FIGURE 7.5

Male and Female Lung Cancer Mortality Rates, 1983–1987 (*U. S. average = 46.4)

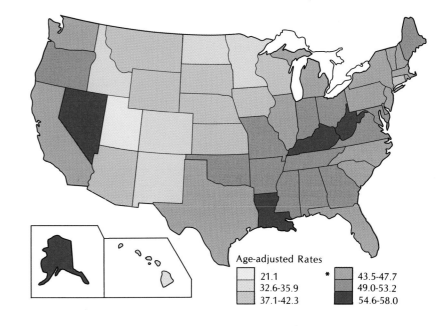

1980s occurred in Kentucky, West Virginia, and Maryland. Some northeastern states also reported average to higher-than-average rates. While the female lung cancer mortality rate for the period 1983–1987 was much more than 10 times the rate for women in the 1930–1932 period, the male lung cancer mortality rate was 3 times higher than the female rate during the 1980s.

During the period 1983–1987, the average male lung cancer mortality rate per 100,000 persons was 73.9. This figure was 25 times higher than the rate for the 1930–1932 period. In addition, regional patterns of clustering were substantially different for male mortality during the 1983–1987 period. The male lung cancer

pattern in 1983–1987 is shown in Figure 7.7. The highest concentrations of male lung cancer mortality during the mid-1980s occurred in the southeastern United States. A high-lung cancer core area included Louisiana, Arkansas, Mississippi, Alabama, Georgia, Kentucky, Tennessee, and Virginia. Higher-than-average male lung cancer mortality rates were also reported in states on the fringe of this core area, including Florida, Texas, Oklahoma, Missouri, Illinois, Indiana, Ohio, North Carolina, South Carolina, and Maryland. Thus, while the Southeast had some of the lowest lung cancer mortality rates during the 1930s, it had the highest rates during the 1980s. Central parts of the United

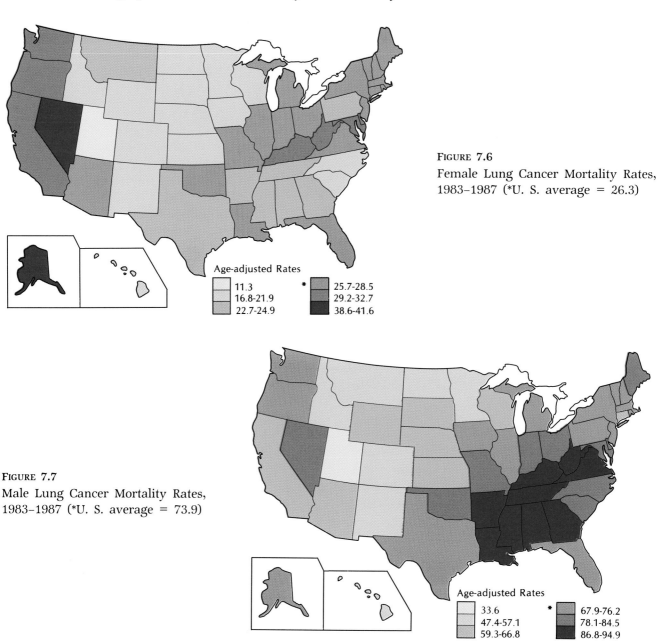

FIGURE 7.6
Female Lung Cancer Mortality Rates, 1983–1987 (*U. S. average = 26.3)

Age-adjusted Rates

11.3	* 25.7-28.5
16.8-21.9	29.2-32.7
22.7-24.9	38.6-41.6

FIGURE 7.7
Male Lung Cancer Mortality Rates, 1983–1987 (*U. S. average = 73.9)

Age-adjusted Rates

33.6	* 67.9-76.2
47.4-57.1	78.1-84.5
59.3-66.8	86.8-94.9

States continued to report lower-than-average lung cancer mortality rates for males, with Utah reporting the lowest rate.

Without a doubt, the accelerated lung cancer mortality rates in the United States among both men and women, and particularly among men, reflect some present-day health problems that are directly attributable to tobacco consumption. In spite of antismoking campaigns that have been conducted both by the United States government and by many private foundations, the lung cancer mortality problem is lingering and, indeed, becoming increasingly worse in the Southeast.

Cultural, behavioral and economic circumstances all appear to be contributing to this regional problem. A geographical perspective on these contributory factors may be obtained by examining Figures 7.8 and 7.9. Figure 7.8 shows a strong regional cluster of tobacco-producing states. The heaviest concentration of tobacco production in the United States occurs in North Carolina, Kentucky, South Carolina, Tennessee, and Virginia. When the pattern in Figure 7.8 is compared to that in Figure 7.9, a direct association can be made. Note that many states with either no clean indoor air laws or only nominal ordinances are mostly concentrated in the Southeast and heavily overlap with tobacco production. While some northeastern manufacturing states, such as New Jersey and New York, have enacted very extensive clean indoor air laws, quite the opposite is true in the Deep South. Even California,

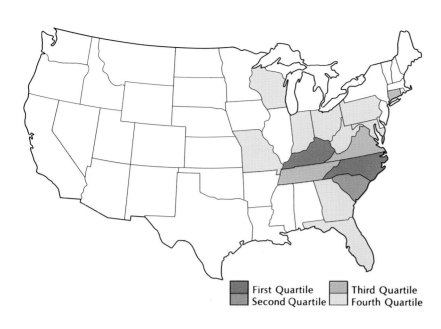

FIGURE 7.8

Tobacco Producing States in 1989 (Tobacco as a percentage of total agricultural receipts)

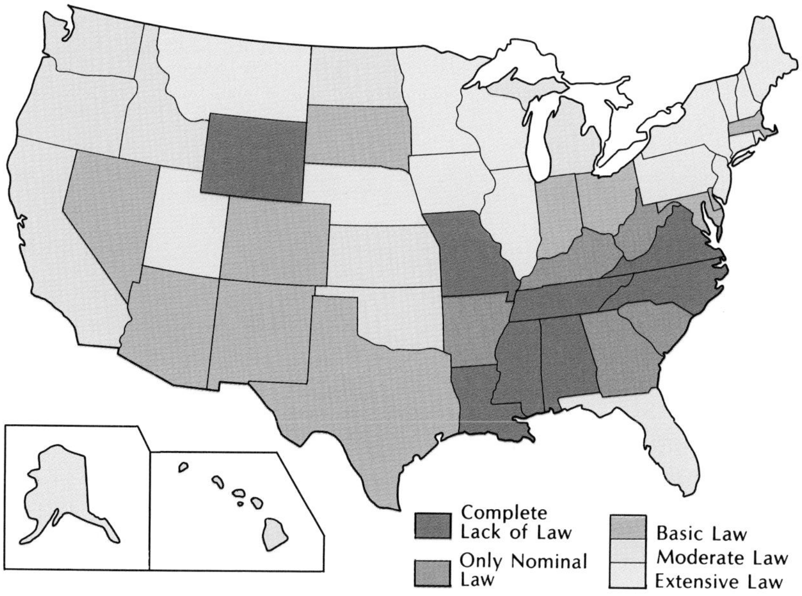

First Quartile   Third Quartile
Second Quartile   Fourth Quartile

FIGURE 7.9

States with and without Clean Indoor Air Laws in 1989

Complete Lack of Law   Basic Law
Only Nominal Law   Moderate Law
Extensive Law

noted for strong support of environmental issues, does not have antismoking laws as strong as those of the upper Midwest and the Northeast. In some of the tobacco-producing states, economic interests have definitely inhibited the enactment of clean indoor air laws. Though it is clear that even secondhand smoke can contribute to lung cancer, it is still difficult to find no-smoking sections in many restaurants in the South. The failure to enact such laws indirectly contributes to social acceptance of smoking and other tobacco use in general, particularly among young persons.

The American Cancer Society has annually sponsored "The Great American Smokeout" since the late 1970s. The purpose of this program is to encourage smokers to at least refrain from tobacco use for 24 continuous hours. As indicated by the patterns shown in Figure 7.9 regarding enactment of clean indoor air laws, many state legislatures have taken this program and similar activities seriously.

A problem that still exists, however, is that increasing numbers of persons of high school age have become regular smokers during recent years. A major national health objective is to reduce the initiation of smoking by young people in the year 2000 to no more than 15 percent who become regular smokers by age 20. Specific measures that can be used to obtain this objective, particularly in high schools, include implementation of strong health education programs on hazards related to tobacco consumption, establishment of completely tobacco-free environments in schools, and continued enactment and enforcement of laws prohibiting the sale and distribution of tobacco to minors. Two additional measures that will assist in attaining this goal include the complete elimination of tobacco product advertising in areas frequented by young people and the enactment of strong clean indoor air laws in all 50 states. The parts of the country that seem to require increased attention in order to meet these goals include the West Coast and the Southeast.

In part, the strongly pronounced regional cluster of male lung cancer deaths during the mid-1980s in the Southeast seems to overshadow the problem among females. As previously indicated, even though the female lung cancer mortality rate in the United States during recent years has been about one-third the male rate, it is still an increasing problem.

BREAST CANCER

Ancient Egyptians described breast cancer and its treatment some 5,000 years ago, and Indian writings dating to 2000 B.C. as well as the cuneiform tablets of Assyria record the occurrence of breast cancer. While no general treatment was described in Egypt, one reported case was cauterized with a hot stick. In India, treatment of breast tumors consisted of surgical removal of the tumor, cauterization, and the ingestion of arsenic compounds. By the fifth century B.C., the Greeks also were treating breast cancer by surgery but were discouraged by the number of women who subsequently died from the surgery, from infection, and from the spreading of the cancer. As a result, treatment of "hidden" (nonulcerative) breast cancer was discouraged. However, in the first and second centuries A.D. the Romans regularly performed extensive surgery for breast cancer, including removal of the pectoral (chest) muscles. As with so many aspects of medicine and science, during the Middle Ages there was little change in procedures for dealing with breast cancer. Monks in Europe did record and transmit limited descriptions of the surgical and cautery procedures used, but these were only sketchy summaries.

Surgery for breast cancer was reintroduced into Western culture during the Renaissance, beginning in 1453. For several centuries, there was considerable debate about the extent to which tumors and surrounding tissue should be surgically removed. By the seventeenth century, surgeons generally abstained from operating when large areas of the breast were affected. Alternate treatments included the application of warm goose or duck blood and a mixture of crawfish boiled in ass milk. Well into the nineteenth century, nightshade (such as the poisonous belladonna plant) and impure zinc oxide were applied locally to the hard lumps and ulcers. Also, applications of caustic agents such as lime arsenic and sandrak, which caused reactions similar to the application of fire (cautery), were frequent. Women were also purged with various emetics or bled to limit the production of black bile which was believed to build up in their breasts. Specific diets were recommended, notably avoidance of "hot" (spicy) foods. As late as 1924 a quack in Amsterdam was convicted of having split open a live puppy to apply it to a breast cancer. This "treatment" can be traced to a mid-sixteenth century practice recommended by a surgeon to a French king. In another treatment, women were told to place live toads on their breasts; the theory was that the toads would "suck out" the cancer poison, become overwhelmed by it, and die of convulsions.

Etiology

According to most modern scientists, *cancer* is a genetic disease at the cellular level. Uncontrolled cellular growth is induced by a reactive carcinogenic molecule or another substance (a virus, for example) that transforms molecules into carcinogens. Breast cancer, a complicated form of the disease, is attributed to several phenomena, including genetics; hormone imbalance; extraneous factors such as viruses; diet; obesity; and so-called environmental circumstances such as chemicals in food, drinking water and/or air pollution. The disease seems usually to start with specific focal points and to subsequently spread. Stages of development thus include small, operable tumors; somewhat larger, but still possibly operable tumors; still larger tumors but still with no spread of the disease to other parts of the body; and finally, widespread or systemic cancer. When the last stage is diagnosed clinically, death can take place within 3 to 4 years.

Over the years, extensive research has been undertaken with respect to breast cancer, and epidemiological studies have shown a variety of positive agents. Genetic aspects of the disease cannot be ignored, because quite often women with close relatives who have had breast cancer also develop the disorder. Epidemiologists have also made strong associations between breast cancer and child bearing late in life. Still other researchers have found that early childbearing combined with extensive breast-feeding tends to lower the risk of breast cancer. Genetic aspects of the disease also appear to be somewhat mysterious. Japanese female breast cancer has been studied extensively, and in mainland Japan the rate is fairly low by international standards; however, Japanese women who move to the United States and live here for an extensive period of time eventually develop rates of breast cancer not substantially different from those of Caucasian Americans. There are also several interesting theories in the area of viral carcinogenesis, the most serious of which pertain to long-term or latent viruses that may be activated by some form of immunological weakening of one's system. The viral hypothesis will have to receive further scientific support in order to be widely accepted by the medical community.

Macroscale Geographic Comparisons

One of the most intriguing hypotheses emerging from international comparisons of breast cancer mortality rates centers on different levels of animal fat consumption. This hypothesis has been around since the late 1960s and the early 1970s. The statistical relationship between breast cancer mortality and animal fat intake is fairly strong. For example, total fat intake is substantially lower in Japan than that in the United States, which explains the variable rates between Japanese and Japanese-American women. Countries with fairly high breast cancer mortality rates and high proportions of animal fat intake include Greece, Spain, Poland, Portugal, Italy, and Austria. There are also higher-than-average international rates in the United States, Canada, Switzerland, France, The Netherlands, Belgium, Denmark, New Zealand, and Germany. Interesting studies of women of varied geographical origins who had migrated to Israel showed higher rates among women of European origin and lower rates among women from some sections of Africa and from other parts of the Middle East.

Another international aspect of breast cancer mortality is that it has been steadily, though slowly, on the increase since about the mid-1950s. According to the U.S. Public Health Service, Centers for Disease Control, premature mortality due to breast cancer in the United States will continue to increase during the 1990s and the first decade of the twenty-first century, and will probably peak after about the year 2010. The substantial increase in breast cancer in the United States has been attributed to the continuing increase in the ratio of women to men because women are living longer; thus more women survive into the higher-cancer-risk years. The importance of the disease in the United States can be understood when one realizes that, by the late 1980s, 20 percent of cancer deaths in women were due to breast cancer. The National Cancer Insti-

tute also reports that the incidence of breast cancer in younger women (25 to 44 years of age) is now on the increase.

Geographic Variations within the United States

Figures 7.10 to 7.12 present a series of maps depicting variable numbers of deaths due to breast cancer per 100,000 women in the United States for the period 1930–1932 and the years 1950 and 1986. These maps demonstrate that some parts of the country have maintained essentially the same incidence of breast cancer during this century. Other regions have reported much change. At the beginning of the Depression, the national average was 19.2 deaths per 100,000 females. States with the highest incidence of female breast cancer during the early 1930s were California, Minnesota, New York, Maryland, New Jersey, Delaware, Connecticut, Massachusetts, and Rhode Island. Most states in the northwestern United States and in the traditional northeastern manufacturing belt had rates of breast cancer mortality that were near the average or somewhat above. In contrast, the parts of the country with the lowest incidence of breast cancer included large parts of the Hispanic Southwest (excluding southern California); some Great Plains states, including the Dakotas, Kansas, and Oklahoma; and most of the southeastern United States.

The national average for breast cancer deaths per 100,000 females by 1950 was 22.5. The southern and southwestern portions of the United States had not changed drastically during the Depression and World War II. In other words, the Southeast as well as the Hispanic sections of the Southwest continued to have some of the lowest breast cancer mortality rates. Large portions of the Northeast continued to report some of the highest rates. In 1950, rates appeared to be the highest in most of New England as well as in New York, Pennsylvania, New Jersey, Maryland, and Delaware. There were also mostly higher than average rates in the midwestern sections of the manufacturing belt as well as in some parts of the upper Midwest. California and Oregon, along with Colorado, showed higher-than-average rates by 1950, while some of the lowest rates showed up in Wyoming and Nevada.

The pattern of incidence of female breast cancer remained somewhat the same by the late 1980s, but there were some changes in the incidence of the disease in western parts of the United States. By the late 1980s, the highest concentrations of breast cancer mortality were still located primarily in the Northeast. Northeastern states that had been near average or somewhat higher than average during the 1930s and

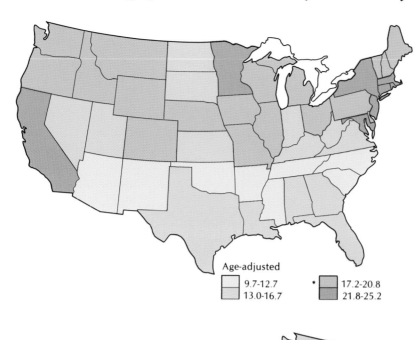

FIGURE 7.10
Female Breast Cancer Mortality Rates, 1930–1932 (*U. S. average = 19.2)

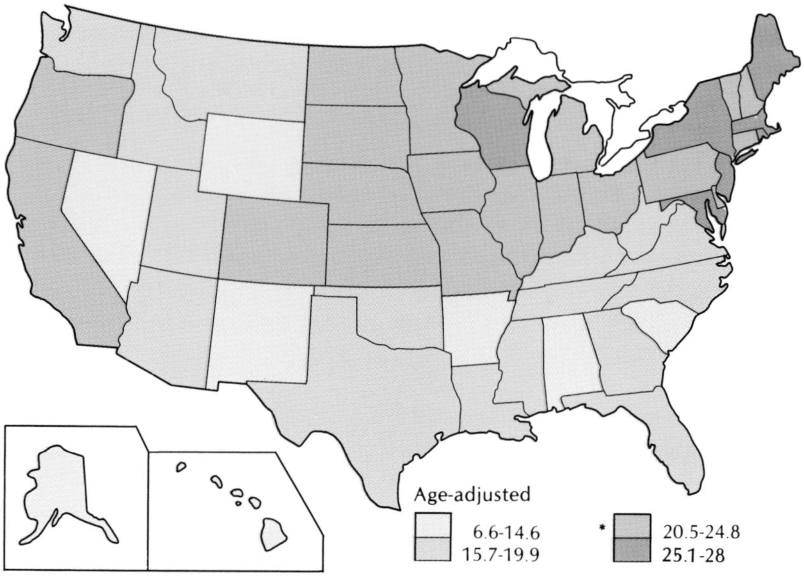

FIGURE 7.11
Female Breast Cancer Mortality Rates, 1950 (*U. S. average = 22.5)

1950s really stood out as being substantially above average by the late 1980s. In addition, Wyoming, Montana, and South Dakota began to show higher-than-average rates, along with Nebraska, Kansas and Minnesota, which had periodically had higher-than-average breast cancer mortality rates, but not so high as some northeastern states. Most West Coast states showed average to higher-than-average breast cancer mortality rates by the late 1980s. Once again, in the late 1980s, the Hispanic Southwest and the South continued to report breast cancer mortality rates below the national average.

In general, patterns of geographic similarities and differences in breast cancer mortality during most of the twentieth century in the United States have reflected aspects of the disease that had been previously pointed out in many studies of breast cancer. For ex-

ample, as the incidence of breast cancer has increased in most parts of the world during the twentieth century, it has also increased in the United States. The interesting association between animal fat intake and breast cancer mortality cannot be taken lightly, given evidence that as some countries of the world become more industrialized and presumably more "Westernized," dietary practices also depart from traditional protein intake and include increased amounts of animal fat. In addition, age continues to be a factor in the incidence of breast cancer worldwide and in the United States, as women begin to live longer.

A new case of breast cancer is discovered in the United States every 15 minutes. By 1991, there may be close to 150,000 new cases of the disease, as compared to about 68,000 new cases in 1965. Many public health agencies report that percentages of American women

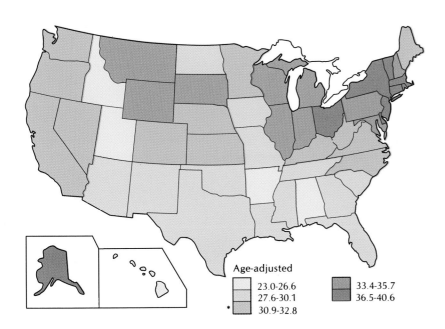

Age-adjusted

23.0-26.6	33.4-35.7
27.6-30.1	36.5-40.6
* 30.9-32.8	

who had had screening mammograms increased substantially during the late 1980s and early 1990s. Some of these increased numbers of new cases can be attributed to early detection in numbers of women above the age of 50 who have had these annual mammogram screenings.

Conclusion

Several factors appear to contribute to differences in the incidence of breast cancer. The first of these is clearly genetic. The genetic predisposition takes the form of family history: women whose relatives have developed breast cancer have risk factors about 3 times higher than women who do not have family histories of breast cancer. Studies have also indicated that Caucasians are genetically more susceptible to breast cancer than are blacks. However, as more and more black women attain higher socioeconomic status, these differences have tended to decline. Another epidemiological aspect of the disease may be reflected in geographic differences in dietary preferences. Yet another

deals with postmenopausal women who have gone through specific hormonal changes. Some parts of the country have higher concentrations of women in more advanced age groups, creating higher probabilities of adverse hormonal environments. There is some speculation that elderly women on immunosuppressive drugs and women who have been exposed to heavy ionizing radiation also seem to have higher-than-expected rates. Radiation exposure is expected to be a topic of future research.

Other personal and demographic factors that have been linked to one extent or another with risk of breast cancer include various types of obesity, hypertension, and diabetes. Latitudinal banding has been hypothesized: researchers have speculated that higher, colder latitudes have an impact in the form of a higher incidence of breast cancer. Studies that indicate both environmental and genetic causes of breast cancer will continue to be made. From a geographic perspective, the most intriguing association occurs between diet and the incidence of the disease, particularly with regard to migration patterns.

STOMACH CANCER

We turn now to an examination of stomach cancer, a specific type of cancer that has caused far fewer deaths during this century than either breast cancer or lung cancer. During the early part of this century, stomach cancer was a leading cause of death for both men and women, with about 50 percent more men than women perishing from this disorder. It has been estimated that about 60 men and about 50 women per

100,000 population in most large cities were dying of stomach cancer annually around the turn of the century. By 1930, when more consistent and comprehensive statewide statistics were collected and released by federal and private agencies, male stomach cancer death rates were nearly 40 per 100,000 and female rates were almost 30 per 100,000 persons (Figure 7.13 and 7.14).

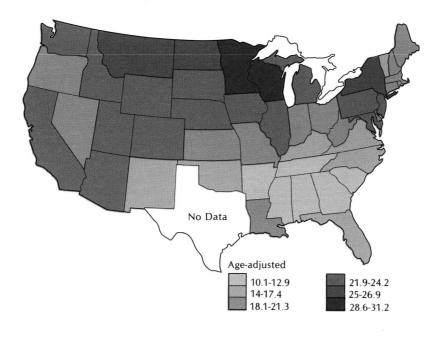

FIGURE 7.13
Male Stomach Cancer Mortality Rates, 1930–1932

No Data

Age-adjusted

10.1-12.9	21.9-24.2
14-17.4	25-26.9
18.1-21.3	28.6-31.2

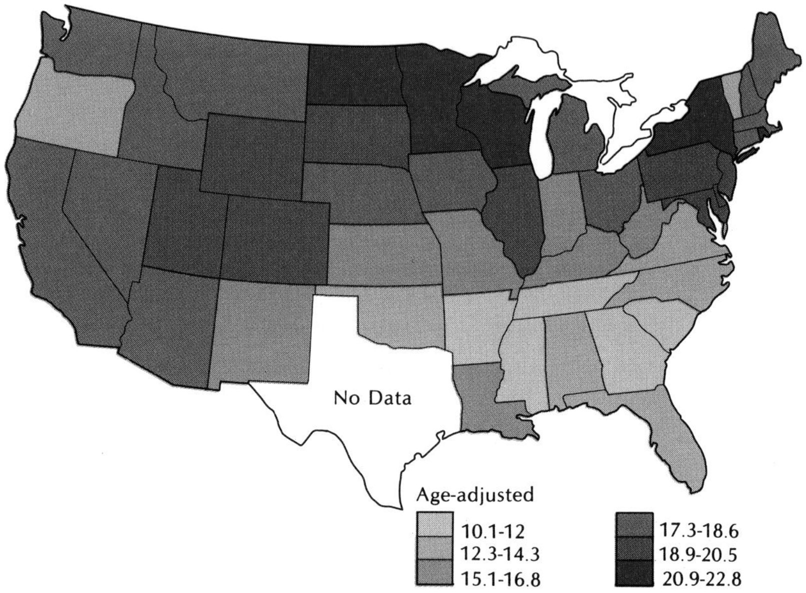

FIGURE 7.14
Female Stomach Cancer Mortality Rates, 1930–1932

No Data

Age-adjusted

10.1-12	17.3-18.6
12.3-14.3	18.9-20.5
15.1-16.8	20.9-22.8

Perhaps more so than many other forms of the disease, stomach cancer rates can be lowered through modification of diet. It has long been known that some specific foods can lead to stomach cancer if consumed over long periods of time on a regular basis. One such example is soy sauce. Stomach cancer rates in Japan have traditionally been higher than those in most other countries due to the quantities of soy sauce regularly consumed. While such regional clusters of high-incidence stomach cancer rates can be explained by dietary habits of certain cultures as well as by individual or group behavior, no single factor has continued to explain the high incidence of stomach cancer over long periods of time in the United States.

Six factors appear to interact in various combinations to contribute to elevated stomach cancer rates, and most of these factors either directly or indirectly pertain to types and quantities of foods consumed. The first factor consists of common food consumption patterns that are directly related to types of regional agricultural production. In other words, environmental conditions in different regions of the United States lead to regional specialization in animal and vegetable agricultural products. Thus, regions that produce large amounts of dairy and beef cattle are characterized by substantial consumption of red meat, sometimes in combination with dairy products. Conversely, parts of the country that produce large amounts of green vegetables but considerably less cattle have very different and often lower patterns of stomach cancer incidence.

The second contributing factor appears to be cultural. As already mentioned, some ethnic groups demonstrate defined behavior patterns with respect to types of food consumed. For decades, many large American cities have been characterized by a wide range of ethnic groups who consume an equally wide variety of foods.

Another factor that affects stomach cancer rates is availability of financial resources. This factor, paradoxically, seems to be related to both very high and very low stomach cancer rates. For example, in some urban areas, foods consumed by poor people consist of fatty and less desirable cuts of meat, with few fresh vegetables. Conversely, in poor agricultural regions the consumption of large quantities of certain kinds of green vegetables has actually led to lower-than-average stomach cancer rates.

Yet another factor which contributes to stomach cancer rates is general economic conditions within regions. It is also possible to show that stomach cancer rates have increased immediately following some periods of economic depression or recession.

A fifth factor that contributes to differences in regional stomach cancer rates is the availability of various kinds of food products. Regional preferences determine what products are grown locally, and availability is also affected by the seasonality of different products and by the cost of shipment over long distances.

Finally, the role of food additives in explaining differences in stomach cancer rates cannot be overlooked. Many of the preservatives and additives found in products on the market in the United States, particularly in the 1970s and the 1980s, have been known to contribute to stomach cancer under controlled experimental conditions. Some additives, in fact, have been on the market for only short periods of time.

None of the contributory factors mentioned above are assumed to be consistent over long periods of time. During the first two decades of this century, both the cities of the United States and the agricultural areas were substantially different from the way they are today. During the Great Depression, when more than one-third of the labor force were unemployed during various periods, proper diet was sometimes secondary to outright survival. In addition, rationing during World War II led to the consumption of some products on a very limited basis. It would be difficult to imagine a large family gathering during the 1990s for a holiday meal at which the main dish was a large cube of roasted canned meat garnished by sliced pineapple, but such a scene was fairly common during the 1940s. Even the post-World War II period was characterized

by inadequate diets on the part of many because of shortages of some commodities, a rapidly growing and migratory population, and adjustments in the agricultural system. In the boom period of the 1960s and the mid-1970s, many foods that previously had been heavily concentrated in only certain regions of the country became widely available. In addition, the completion of a modern interstate highway system led to an even broader distributional network of food products nationally. Within cities, older established ethnic neighborhoods often broke up and populations of subsequent generations were dispersed to a wide range of suburban and nonurban locations.

Many factors of modern society, educational programs, and public awareness of possible problems resulting from some food additives have contributed to a substantial decline in stomach cancer rates over the past sixty years. The 1960 stomach cancer rate for males was about 17 per 100,000 persons, or less than half that of 1930. By 1990, the male stomach cancer rate was half that of 1960. A similar trend can be identified among females. The 1960 female stomach cancer rate of about 8 deaths per 100,000 persons was one-third that of 1930, and the 1990 rate was about half that of 1960. Overall, stomach cancer rates for both males and females have declined even as other cancers, such as lung cancer, have increased.

National state-based stomach cancer mortality rate information is published by the National Center for Health Statistics in a fashion that sometimes separates cases and rates by race (i.e., white and nonwhite) and sometimes by set. Data are available for the period 1950–1979, by decade and separated into male and female categories. The period 1983–1987 has been averaged by race, but unfortunately not by sex. The sequence of maps shown in Figures 7.15 to 7.17 gives some indication of regional patterns of variation for stomach cancer in the United States during the post-World War II period, depending upon the nature of the available information.

Geographic Patterns in Mortality Rates

White Males

1950–1979. The maps in Figures 7.15 to 7.17 depict both changes and consistencies in the pattern of white male stomach cancer mortality in the United States during the 1950s, the 1960s, and the 1970s. Note the pattern in Figure 7.15 for the period 1950–1959. Clearly, the heaviest concentrations of male stomach cancer during the 1950s were in the northern tier of states extending from east to west across much of the

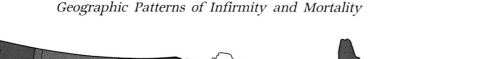

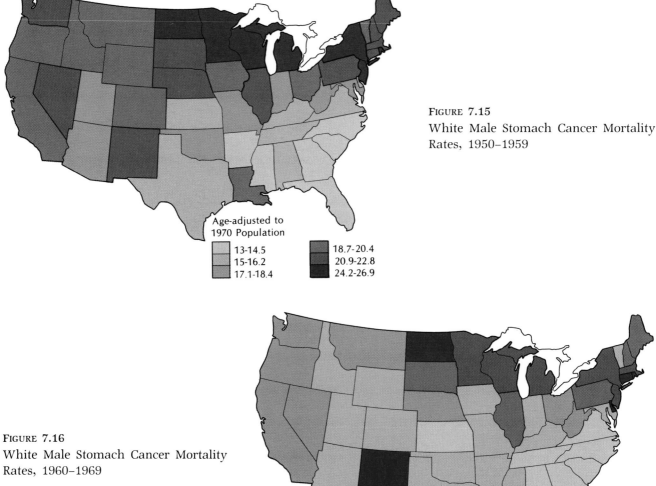

FIGURE 7.15
White Male Stomach Cancer Mortality
Rates, 1950–1959

Age-adjusted to
1970 Population

13-14.5	18.7-20.4
15-16.2	20.9-22.8
17.1-18.4	24.2-26.9

FIGURE 7.16
White Male Stomach Cancer Mortality
Rates, 1960–1969

Age-adjusted

8.4-10	13.8-14.7
10.4-11.7	15.3-16.3
12.2-13.4	16.7-18.4

Canadian border. This area is, of course, a dairy belt. Other parts of the western United States known for cattle ranching also were characterized by higher-than-average rates of stomach cancer. It is quite interesting to note in the pattern of the Mississippi Delta area that Louisiana stood out with higher-than-average white male stomach cancer mortality rates during the 1950s. This pattern might be attributed to the spicy Cajun food that is often eaten in this area.

By the 1960s the white male stomach cancer mortality rate was also very low in the Southeast (Figure 7.16). As in the 1950s, most of the concentrations of higher-than-average white male stomach mortality rates for the 1960s were in the northern parts of the country. However, New Mexico stood out with excep-

tionally high mortality rates, along with Connecticut. The general North-South regional distinctions continued into the 1970s. The pattern shown in Figure 7.17 for the 1970–1979 time frame again indicated an extensive area along the Canadian border states as well as in the northeastern parts of the United States with higher-than-average white male stomach cancer mortality rates. Once again during the 1970s, the Southeast reported the lowest regional rates of white male stomach cancer mortality.

White Females

1950–1979. Regional differences in the incidence of white female stomach cancer mortality during the

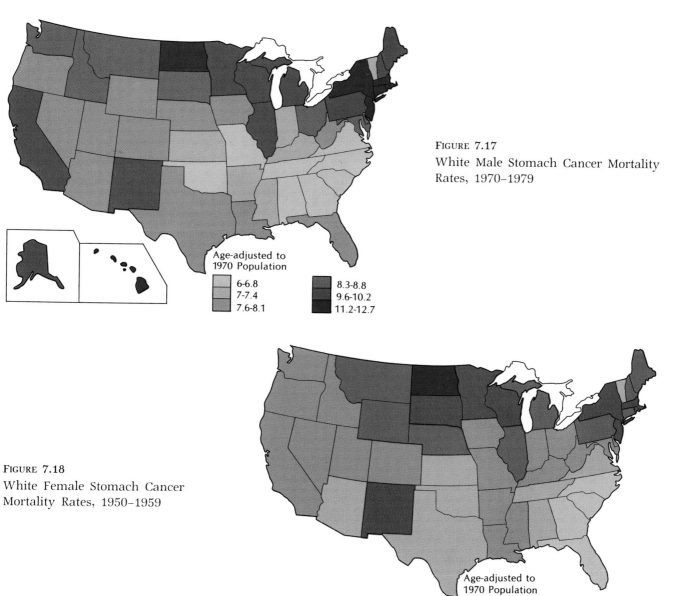

FIGURE 7.17
White Male Stomach Cancer Mortality Rates, 1970–1979

Age-adjusted to 1970 Population

6-6.8	8.3-8.8
7-7.4	9.6-10.2
7.6-8.1	11.2-12.7

FIGURE 7.18
White Female Stomach Cancer Mortality Rates, 1950–1959

Age-adjusted to 1970 Population

6.8-7.4	10.8-11.9
7.9-8.8	12.5-14.1
9.1-10.5	17

post-World War II period were somewhat similar to male patterns. Figures 7.18 to 7.20 show white female stomach cancer mortality patterns during the periods 1950–1959, 1960–1969, and 1970–1979, respectively. Patterns are somewhat similar for all these decades. The pattern during the 1950s, as depicted in Figure 7.18, for example, shows a pattern of highest-incidence states clustered in the northern Great Plains areas as well as in sections of the northeastern dairy belt and parts of New England and New Jersey. New Mexico also stood out during the late 1950s as reporting higher-than-average white female stomach cancer mortality rates. The lowest regional concentrations were, once again, in the Southeast. The 1950s pattern of white female stomach cancer mortality held up and

continued through the 1960s. The pattern shown in Figure 7.19 for the period 1960–1969 shows that higher-than-average rates for white females occurred consistently in the upper Great Plains and the midwestern dairy belt, as well as in New York, New Jersey, and the New England states. Once again, New Mexico stood out, almost isolated in the Southwest, as a state with higher-than-average white female stomach cancer mortality. The southeastern parts of the United States once again reported the lowest regional clustering. Regional clustering in the 1970s continued to be similar to that of the previous two decades, with some subtle differences. The upper Midwest was still characterized by higher-than-average rates, along with parts of the Northeast and New Mexico. Also, the Southeast

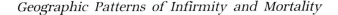

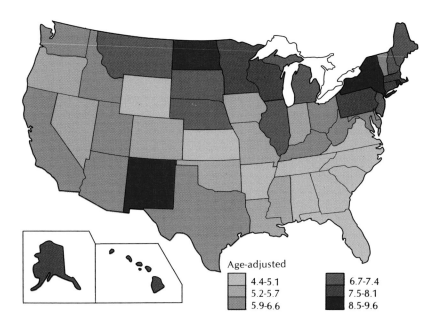

FIGURE 7.19
White Female Stomach Cancer
Mortality Rates, 1960–1969

FIGURE 7.20
White Female Stomach Cancer
Mortality Rates, 1970–1979

continued to report lower-than-average rates. By the 1970s, however, California began to report white female stomach cancer mortality rates at about the national average. Figure 7.17, which shows white male stomach cancer mortality for the 1970s, also indicates some elevated white male stomach cancer mortality rates in California for the first time.

Black Males

1950–1979. Regional differences in black male stomach cancer mortality rates during the 1950s, the 1960s, and the 1970s (Figures 7.21 to 7.23) are characterized by variable regional concentrations. Black male stomach cancer mortality rates are shown in Figure 7.21 for the period 1950–1959. States with higher-than-average black male stomach cancer mortality rates during the 1950s were quite widespread. While overall black male stomach cancer mortality rates during the 1950s were almost twice as high as white rates, the only significant cluster consisted of Pennsylvania, New Jersey, New York, and Connecticut. Other than this pocket in the Northeast and a fairly high rate reported for New Hampshire (a state with a limited black population), states with higher-than-average rates were somewhat scattered. As with whites, Louisiana did stand out as a state with higher-than-average rates during the 1950s. In a pattern similar to that of white male stomach cancer mortality rates, the region of the country with the concentration of lowest reporting was the Southeast.

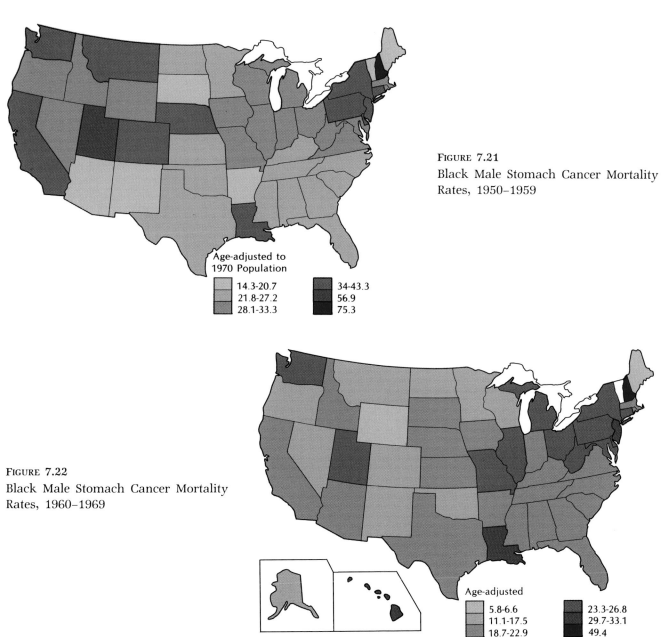

FIGURE 7.21
Black Male Stomach Cancer Mortality
Rates, 1950–1959

Age-adjusted to
1970 Population

14.3-20.7	34-43.3
21.8-27.2	56.9
28.1-33.3	75.3

FIGURE 7.22
Black Male Stomach Cancer Mortality
Rates, 1960–1969

Age-adjusted

5.8-6.6	23.3-26.8
11.1-17.5	29.7-33.1
18.7-22.9	49.4

By the 1960s (Figure 7.22), black male stomach cancer mortality rates were a little lower than during the 1950s, with an average of about 20 per 100,000. Concentrations were more localized in the northeastern parts of the country. Louisiana, along with New Hampshire, stood out once again, with very high black male stomach cancer mortality rates. The other major cluster was in the manufacturing belt in the Northeast. Though the Southeast continued to report rates at or below average, it was clear that black male stomach cancer mortality rates were on the increase in that area. The pattern for black male stomach cancer mortality during the 1970s was characterized by yet another change (Figure 7.23). By the 1970–1979 period, the highest concentrations were in states east of the Mississippi River. Both the Southeast and the Northeast had been characterized by increases during the 1970s. Whatever the reason for this major regional shift in black male stomach cancer mortality rates, the relative differences between the East and the West became quite striking, as the pattern, shifted from one of little focus to one of heavier concentration, even with lower rates, by the end of the 1970s.

Black Females

1950–1979. The distributional patterns for black female stomach cancer mortality rates during the 1950s, the 1960s, and the 1970s are shown in Figures 7.24 to 7.26. During these three decades, there was no single

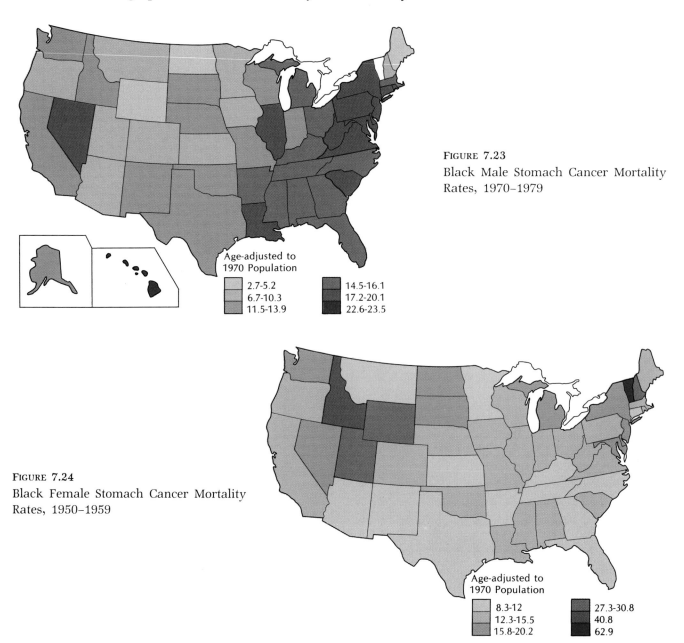

FIGURE 7.23
Black Male Stomach Cancer Mortality
Rates, 1970–1979

FIGURE 7.24
Black Female Stomach Cancer Mortality
Rates, 1950–1959

large cluster of higher-than-average black female stomach cancer mortality; instead, states that were characterized by higher-than-average rates were quite widespread. However, there was some indication by the 1970s that a regional shift had begun, wherein parts of the United States east of the Mississippi had generally started to report somewhat higher-than-average black female stomach cancer mortality rates. This aspect was somewhat offset by some higher concentrations of these rates in the northwestern parts of the country during the 1970s.

Overall Mortality Rates

The 1980s. As previously mentioned, available information from the U.S. Public Health Service, National Center for Health Statistics, for stomach cancer mortality during the 1980s is somewhat different from the information available for previous decades. Figures 7.27 to 7.29 show stomach cancer mortality distributions for the period 1983–1987, age-adjusted to the 1970 population. The pattern shown in Figure 7.27 includes the entire U.S. population, both male and female, including all racial groups. Given that the overall stomach cancer mortality rate during the 1980s was less than one-tenth that of the 1930s, it is not surprising to discover that there was no strong pattern of regional concentration of stomach cancer mortality, other than some residual clustering in and around Pennsylvania, New York, New Jersey, and Connecticut. Such a pattern is an indication of a disease on the decline. States with higher-than-average rates during the 1980s were as

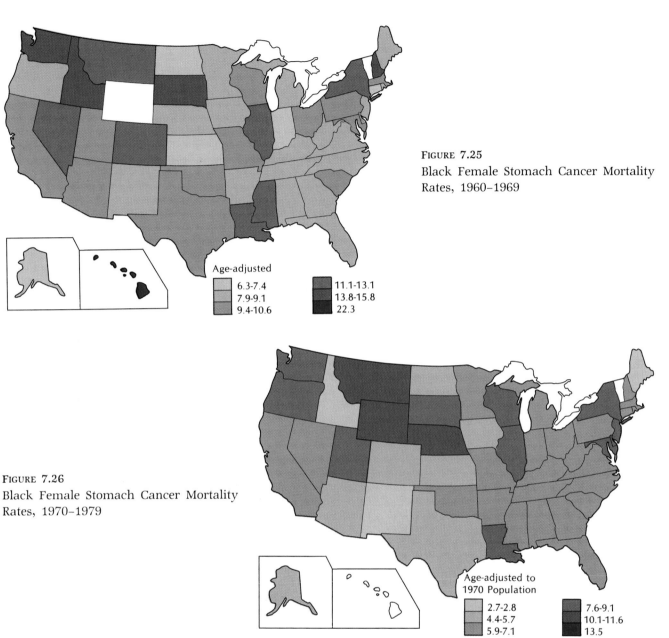

FIGURE 7.25
Black Female Stomach Cancer Mortality
Rates, 1960–1969

Age-adjusted
6.3-7.4
7.9-9.1
9.4-10.6
11.1-13.1
13.8-15.8
22.3

FIGURE 7.26
Black Female Stomach Cancer Mortality
Rates, 1970–1979

Age-adjusted to
1970 Population
2.7-2.8
4.4-5.7
5.9-7.1
7.6-9.1
10.1-11.6
13.5

widespread as North Dakota, California, New Mexico, Illinois, Louisiana, and South Carolina. The Southeast seemed to have lost its lower regional ranking from earlier periods to the central Great Plains region; however, overall rates during the 1980s were substantially lower than in previous decades.

Some regional patterns of concentration are noticed when black and white populations are separated. The distribution shown in Figure 7.28 consists of reporting for white male and white female stomach cancer mortality during the 1980s. The pattern of higher-than-average concentrations along the Canadian border stood out once again, along with the familiar northeastern cluster. The Southeast, however, was more complex, with more variable patterns than those that had existed during previous decades. In addition, Cali-

fornia, Nevada, and New Mexico stood out, showing higher than average rates during the 1980s, along with Florida. The populations of many of the Sunbelt states had changed drastically during the 1980s because of increased migrations of retired persons from other parts of the country, especially the Northeast. It should be expected that many cases of male and female stomach cancer mortality could be more directly attributed to behavioral and dietary customs associated with these persons' regions of origin.

By the 1980s, there also appears to have been an East-West differentiation with regard to black stomach cancer mortality in the United States (Figure 7.29). Many western states simply had no cases to report. However, Washington and Minnesota stood out as the states with the highest black male and female stomach

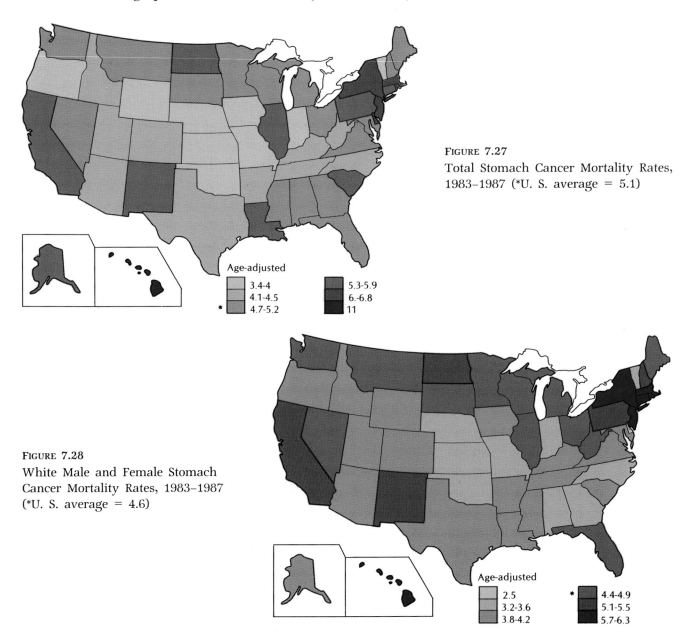

FIGURE 7.27
Total Stomach Cancer Mortality Rates,
1983–1987 (*U. S. average = 5.1)

Age-adjusted

3.4-4		5.3-5.9	
4.1-4.5		6.-6.8	
* 4.7-5.2		11	

FIGURE 7.28
White Male and Female Stomach
Cancer Mortality Rates, 1983–1987
(*U. S. average = 4.6)

Age-adjusted

2.5		* 4.4-4.9	
3.2-3.6		5.1-5.5	
3.8-4.2		5.7-6.3	

cancer mortality rates during the 1980s. Generally, there was more clustering of higher-than-average states in the western United States than in the eastern United States. Once again, changes in dietary patterns as well as regional migration networks contributed to some change in the overall patterns of stomach cancer mortality in the United States.

It is encouraging to note that, unlike lung cancer in both men and women, and also unlike breast cancer in females, stomach cancer mortality within the United States is on the decline. In spite of the decreases, how-ever, black populations, generally characterized as having lower incomes than whites in many parts of the country and hence as being disadvantaged, are also characterized by higher-than-average stomach cancer mortality rates. In addition, there does appear to be an East-West differentiation with regard to the black population. By contrast, a residual North-South distinction remains with regard to the white popula-tion of the country, although these differences appear to be not so substantial as they were during earlier decades.

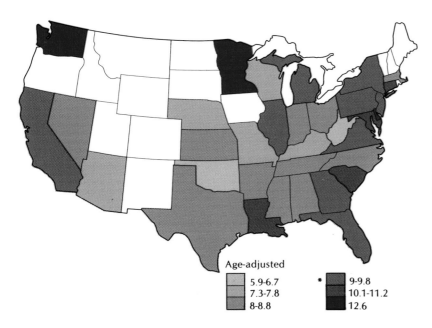

FIGURE 7.29
Black Male and Female Stomach Cancer Mortality Rates, 1983–1987 (*U. S. average = 9.1)

8

Infant Mortality

Infant mortality is one of the most widely used general indices of health in the United States and other countries. It is defined as the number of infant deaths (that is, deaths among children under 1 year of age) per 1,000 live births. The causes of infant mortality are many and complex. A number of general factors have been identified as contributing to observed and changing patterns of infant mortality rates. These include medicine and public health, maternal and infant care, availability and accessibility of medical facilities, and general economic and environmental conditions. Because of the wide range of factors or influences on infant mortality, the rate is often used as a general indicator of the social and economic development of an area, a region, or a nation. However, the number, complexity, and variable interaction of these factors makes it difficult to pinpoint specific change agents. Also, one must be cautious in making strict comparisons and generalizations, especially on the international level.

The twentieth century has witnessed significant changes in the infant mortality rate, and many of these changes can be attributed to the evolution of medicine, public health, and society in the United States. Similarly, geographic differences in infant mortality rates in the United States may be attributed to differences in these factors from place to place.

Detailed consideration of changes in trends and patterns in infant mortality is restricted to the period from the mid-1930s to the early 1990s, primarily because information on both births and deaths is needed to calculate the infant mortality rate. These data for the United States as a whole have been available only since 1933,

the first year in which all states were included in both the Birth Registration Area and the Death Registration Area. A discussion of the evolution of the Death Registration Area, which was first established in 1900, was presented in Chapter 1. The Birth Registration Area was established by the Bureau of the Census in 1915, comprising ten states and the District of Columbia in which the registration of live births was relatively complete. Other states were periodically added to the area, as they met the minimum requirement of 90 percent completeness of birth registration. Generally the states that were added late had comparatively high infant mortality rates. It was not until 1950, when 98 percent of live births in the United States were being registered, that the problem of incompleteness of U.S. birth registration could be dismissed as inconsequential. Data from Birth Registration Area states and from major city estimates of infant mortality rates for the United States are available from 1915.

Mortality Trends

Mortality during the first year of life was fairly common in the United States in the early part of the twentieth century (Figure 8.1). Although precise data are not available, the infant mortality rate in 1915 was estimated to be about 100 per 1,000 live births. In other words, about 10 percent of newborns died before reaching the age of 12 months. While this is a very high mortality rate, it must be recognized that rates of 150 infant deaths per 1,000 live births had been common throughout the United States and much of Europe during the nineteenth century. Even in the early part of the twentieth century, infant mortality rates of over 100 were common in many of the states and cities for which information was available.

During the influenza epidemic of 1918–1919, the U.S. infant mortality rate actually increased to more than 100 deaths per 1,000 live births. Generally, however, the infant mortality rate has declined throughout the twentieth century. The decline was especially notable between 1915 and 1950. In 1950 the infant mortality rate was approximately 29 per 1,000, or only 29 percent of the 1915 rate. In 1989, the infant mortality rate for the United States—9.8 infant deaths per 1,000 live births—was the lowest final rate ever recorded. However, the infant mortality rate in the United States remained higher than that in some 20 other developed countries. Japan had the lowest infant mortality rate, about 5 deaths per 1,000 live births. For the United States, the most recent rate is about 34 percent of the 1950 infant mortality rate. Between 1915 and 1950 the average annual decrease in infant mortality rates was 2.1 deaths per 1,000 live births. Between 1950 and 1990, the average annual decrease was only 0.5 deaths

per 1,000 live births. The downward trend in overall infant mortality has slowed since the late 1970s. One of the nation's health objectives for the year 2000 is to reduce the infant mortality rate for the total population to below 7 infant deaths per 1,000 live births. Thus, the twentieth century has witnessed substantial changes in the infant mortality rate in the United States. The observed changes in the infant mortality rate are matched by substantial changes in the causes of death.

Causes of Death

Generally, the health of an infant may be influenced by factors in the prenatal period as well as in the postnatal period. In other words, the health and nutrition of the mother before and during pregnancy are important determinants of an infant's health status at birth. In the postnatal period, from birth to age 12 months, the newborn child's health is affected by environmental influences such as housing, nutrition, and other living conditions, as well as by infectious and parasitic diseases. In addition, the infant is at risk from condi-

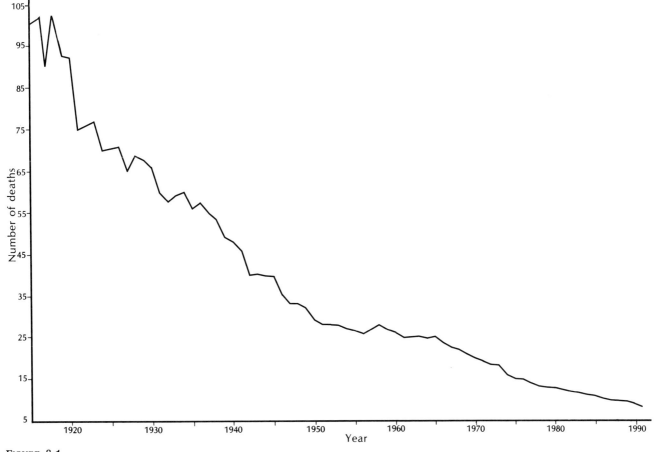

FIGURE 8.1
Infant Deaths per 1,000 Live Births, 1915–1991

tions which have developed in the womb or at birth (congenital defects).

In 1900, though microbial diseases such as pertussis (whooping cough), measles, and tuberculosis were listed, the predominant causes of death among infants were infective and parasitic diseases, influenza and pneumonia, and infections of the digestive system. A small percentage of infant deaths were also usually attributed to premature birth and injury at birth. The smallest percentage were attributed to congenital malformations.

By 1989, in contrast, congenital malformations were the leading cause of death among all infants, accounting for some 21 percent of total deaths. The recently recognized and mysterious sudden infant death syndrome accounted for about 14 percent of the deaths. Ten percent of deaths were attributed to premature birth and low birth weight. In stark contrast to the earlier period, pneumonia and influenza were identified as the least frequent causes of death, together accounting for fewer than 2 percent of infant deaths in 1989. In fact, there has been almost a total elimination of infant infectious diseases (about 2 percent of all infant deaths) and pneumonia and influenza (less than 2 percent) as causes of death during this century. These types of diseases and health conditions have been replaced by disorders related to short gestation period and unspecified but low birth weights. What has contributed to this dramatic change in the causes of infant mortality?

Advances in Medical Care

There were a number of significant developments in medicine in the United States in the early and middle parts of twentieth century. These developments account for some of the substantial reductions in observed infant mortality rates and the changes in causes of death. Of special importance were the development of drugs to combat infectious and parasitic diseases, and the development of vaccines to prevent infection.

Particularly important was the development of a general class of drugs—sulfonamides or sulfa drugs—which are used chiefly in combating infectious disease and bacterial infections, including dysentery (intestinal infection) and pneumonia. These drugs became commonly available in the mid-1930s. In addition, penicillin was described and named in 1929. Its subsequent development as a treatment for many types of bacterial infections was especially important in the fight against pneumonias of many types. It became the primary drug of choice and was instrumental in reducing mortality from influenza and pneumonia.

Advances in Public Health and Social Reform

An analysis of the trends in infant mortality in the United States, however, suggests that major declines were occurring prior to the availability of these medicines. These declines were due to changes in the public health and social reform arenas. In most major cities, milk supplies were being pasturized, visiting nurse services had been developed, and well-baby clinics had been established. Campaigns against illiteracy and promotion of education were also factors. Notable too was the decline in the birth rate from 35 per 100,000 population in 1900 to 18.7 in the late 1920s. Thus, families generally had more resources and time to devote to fewer children. This decline in the birth rate occurred as a tremendous number of people moved to the cities.

In recent years, vaccination and immunization of newly born infants against diseases which threaten their health have become common practices. Among the dangerous childhood diseases against which children are protected are polio, measles (including rubella or German measles), mumps, diphtheria, tetanus (lockjaw), and pertussis. Today it is recommended that children receive their first immunizations against diptheria, tetanus, and pertussis, as well as polio, at the age of 2 months. In addition, health care and welfare programs have been introduced for the poor, as well as health programs directed toward assisting poor mothers and their newborn babies.

Infant mortality has continued the downward trend that was first observed in the late nineteenth century. While notable successes have been achieved generally, differences still occur between various population groups. In 1989, the risk of dying within the first year of life was 2.3 times greater for black than for white infants, with significant variations by cause. In any event, past as well as current geographic variations in infant mortality rates may be attributed in part to concentrations of relatively poor, uneducated, and minority populations.

Geographic Patterns in Mortality Rates

On the basis of 1910 Census estimates and information available from the small number of Birth Registration Area states, some inferences may be made about the geographic pattern of infant mortality shortly after the turn of the century. There appears to have been considerable geographic variation in infant mortality among the states as well as a strong geographic pattern (Table 8.1).

TABLE 8.1

Estimated Infant Mortality Rates per 1,000 Live Births in Birth Registration Area States and Selected Other States: 1910

Utah	82	Connecticut	127
Washington	84	Massachusetts	131
Kentucky	88	Pennsylvania	140
Montana	90	Maine	140
California	92	New York	144
Minnesota	92	New Hampshire	146
Ohio	116	New Jersey	149
Michigan	124	Rhode Island	158

According to the estimates in Table 8.1, in 1910 the lowest infant mortality rates, between 82 and 92 deaths per 1,000 births, occurred in western states such as Utah, California, Washington, and Montana. In the more populous and industrial states of the Midwest, such as Ohio and Michigan, the rates were higher, 116 and 128, respectively. The highest infant mortality rates per 1,000 live births occurred in the most densely settled and urbanized states of the northeast, including New York (144), Connecticut (127), New Jersey (149), and Rhode Island (158). However, exceptionally high infant mortality rates also occurred in relatively sparsely settled Maine (140) and New Hampshire (146). Insofar as these estimates can be relied upon, in 1910 there appears to have been a very strong decline in infant mortality rates away from the northeastern states across the Midwest and toward the Far West. Insufficient data were available at the time to make estimates for the states in the Southeast.

Comparative Rates in the United States

1935. By 1935, the national average infant mortality rate had declined to about 56 deaths per 1,000 live births (Figure 8.2). In 1935 there was one major regional concentration of infant mortality in the United States. The region extended from Kentucky, West Virginia, and Maryland southward along the Gulf Coast and across the Deep South from South Carolina to Louisiana. Arkansas was also included in this contiguous region of states with some of the highest infant mortality rates of the period. Infant mortality rates ranged from 66 to 129 deaths per 1,000 live births in states such as Mississippi and South Carolina. It may be speculated that, in large part, these exceptionally high infant mortality rates reflect the general poverty of these states at this time, as well as the large concentrations of black people, the majority of whom were poor, suffered from malnutrition, and were prevented by racial bias from obtaining proper medical care.

In addition to these southern states, Michigan and Illinois also had infant mortality rates ranging from 66 to 79 deaths per 1,000 live births. In part, these high rates may have been due to early migrations of substantial numbers of blacks from the South to work in and around Chicago and Detroit. In these industrial centers too, blacks were faced with discrimination in their attempts to get medical care and were frequently forced to live in inadequate housing.

Moderately high infant mortality rates, from 54 to 64 deaths per 1,000 live births, were found in northeastern states such as New York, Pennsylvania, Ohio, and Indiana. The lowest infant mortality rates, from 41 to 53 deaths per 1,000 live births, were found in midwestern states such as Wisconsin, Minnesota, and Iowa. Low rates extend from Nebraska and Kansas in the Midwest to California and Arizona in the Southwest.

1955. By 1955, after the Great Depression and World War II had ended, great strides had been made in medical care and the obstetrical specialty in medicine had been developed. The average infant mortality rate in the United States was about 26 deaths per 1,000 live births, less than half that reported some 20 years earlier. As shown in Figure 8.3, the geographic patterns in 1955 were not drastically different from the patterns observed in the mid-1930s. With the exception of Kentucky and Tennessee, the southeastern states generally remained the highest in infant mortality, with rates ranging from 27 to 43 deaths per 1,000 live births. Mississippi, with 43, had the highest rate during 1955. Other states with higher-than-average rates included Illinois, Wyoming, New Mexico, and Nevada. Except in Illinois, the high infant mortality rates may have been due in part to the poor health and nutritional status among the large Native American populations living in these states. What appears to have been developing was an intensification and an extension of low infant mortality rates across the South and the Southwest.

Most of the states in New England and in a belt extending from Wisconsin through Utah and Idaho had infant mortality rates ranging from 20 to 22 deaths per 1,000 live births in 1955, below the national average.

1975. By 1975, a general North-South division had developed in infant mortality rates. In a group of southern states stretching across most of the nation from Maryland through Nevada, infant mortality rates were higher than the national average, ranging from 17 to 22 deaths per 1,000 live births. The national average in 1975 was 16 (Figure 8.4). In the Deep South, South Carolina and Mississippi, which had the largest percentages of black populations, were among the states with the highest infant mortality rates. Also in this category

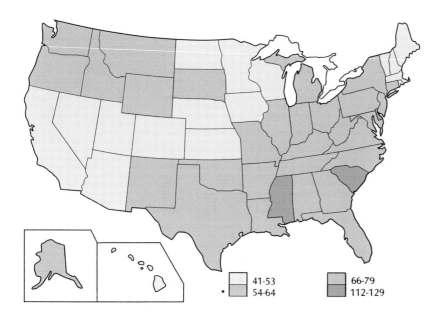

FIGURE 8.2

Infant Deaths per 1,000 Live Births, 1935 (*U. S. average = 56)

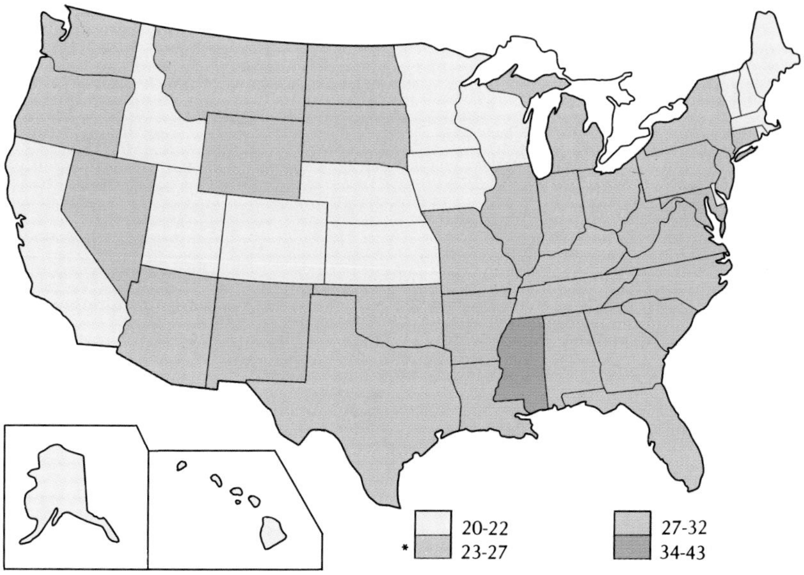

	41-53		66-79
*	54-64		112-129

FIGURE 8.3

Infant Deaths per 1,000 Live Births, 1955 (*U. S. average = 26)

	20-22		27-32
*	23-27		34-43

were New Mexico and Arizona, which had high concentrations of Native Americans and increasing numbers of Hispanics.

Below-average rates were found in only a few states: Idaho and Utah in the West and Minnesota and Iowa in the Midwest. Utah, despite its relatively high percentage of Native Americans, consistently ranked high on all measures of health status. Apparently the lifestyle of the predominantly Mormon population helped to promote physical health. Massachusetts and Connecticut in the Northeast also had lower-than-average infant mortality rates.

1985. Two major changes are apparent when the infant mortality pattern of 1975 is compared to that of 1985. In this 10-year period a number of southern states improved their status with regard to infant mortality. Southern states which had infant mortality rates close to the national average of 11 deaths per 1,000 live births in 1985 included Maryland, West Virginia, and even Mississippi (Figure 8.5). New Mexico, and Arizona had the lowest rankings.

Also significant was the large number of states with below-average infant mortality rates. These states extended from Massachusetts and Rhode Island on the East Coast across the industrial and agricultural Midwest to the Rocky Mountains and Pacific Coast states of Washington, Oregon, and California. It was apparent that improved medical and public health technology for eliminating the threat of infectious diseases through immunization and application of modern medicines, as well as the proliferation of prenatal and

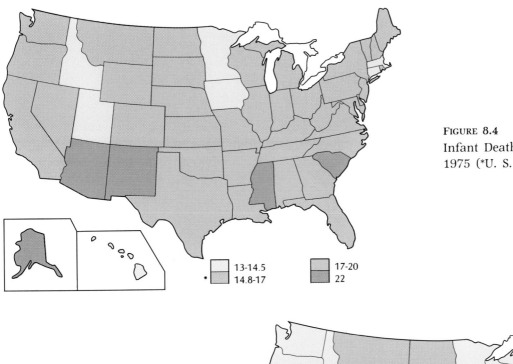

FIGURE 8.4
Infant Deaths per 1,000 Live Births, 1975 (*U. S. average = 16)

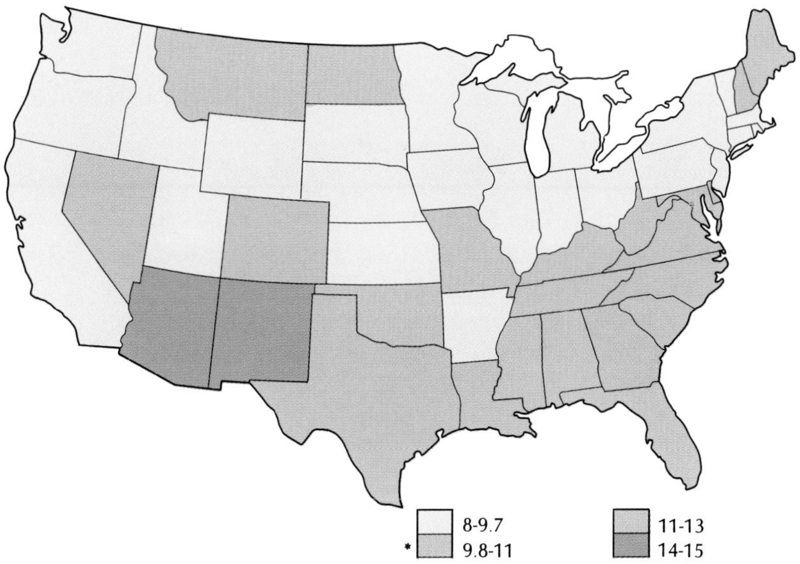

	13-14.5		17-20
*	14.8-17		22

FIGURE 8.5
Infant Deaths per 1,000 Live Births, 1985 (*U. S. average = 10.6)

	8-9.7		11-13
*	9.8-11		14-15

neonatal health programs, had reached a large segment of the population. However, in 1985, as in 1935, there were still large segments of the population, especially the poor and minority populations, which were not benefiting from modern medicine. We examine this phenomenon and other questions below.

Nonwhite-to-White Ratios

In an attempt to develop a better understanding of nonwhite infant mortality patterns in the United States, we have made a geographic comparison of the ratio of nonwhite-to-white infant deaths for selected years from 1935 through 1985, as shown in Figures 8.6 to 8.9. Interestingly, there is almost a complete reversal of geographical patterns over this half-century period.

In 1935 the ratio of nonwhite-to-white infant deaths showed a clear regionalization of highest ratios in the northern Great Plains states, including the Dakotas and Minnesota; in the Pacific Northwest states of Idaho, Oregon, and Washington; and in Nevada, Utah, and Arizona in the Southwest (Figure 8.6). In each of these states, anywhere from 2 to 7 nonwhite infants died for each white infant who died. Most of these states had substantial Native American populations in the 1930s. According to the 1930 census, about two-thirds of the total Native American population (333,000) was living in the states with the most severe infant mortality problems.

As shown in Figure 8.7, the high ratios of nonwhite-to-white infant mortality shifted to the East in the mid-1950s. The highest ratios remained in the upper

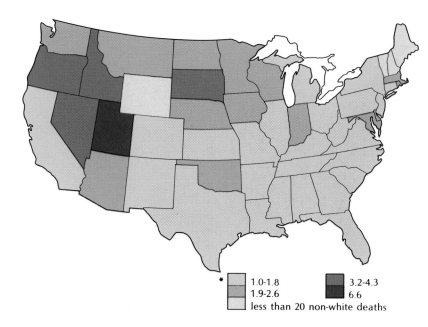

FIGURE 8.6
Infant Mortality: The Number of Non-White Deaths for Every White Death, 1935 (*U. S. average = 1.6)

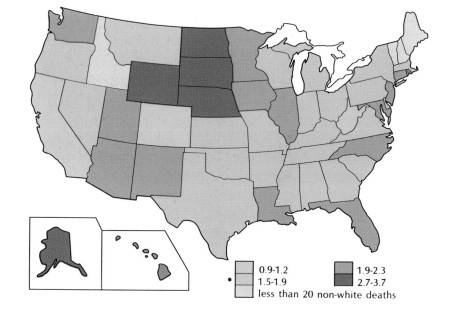

FIGURE 8.7
Infant Mortality: The Number of Non-White Deaths for Every White Death, 1955 (*U. S. average = 1.8)

midwestern states, such as the Dakotas and Nebraska. In these states, between 3 and 4 nonwhite infants died for each white infant who died. Very high nonwhite-to-white ratios were also found in states such as New Jersey, Maryland, and North Carolina on the East Coast and Florida and Louisiana in the Deep South.

In 1955, states with essentially equal ratios of infant mortality (that is, with 1 nonwhite infant dying for each white infant who died) included West Virginia, Colorado, and California. By 1975, the number of states with approximately equal ratios had increased considerably (Figure 8.8). Kentucky, Wisconsin, Oklahoma, Washington, Oregon, California, and Hawaii all had approximately equal ratios, ranging from 1.0 to 1.3.

By 1985, there were more than a dozen states east of the Mississippi River with above-average ratios of nonwhite-to-white infant deaths (Figure 8.9). Included in this category were highly industrialized states such as Michigan, Illinois, Pennsylvania, and New Jersey, as well as more rural states such as Kentucky, Tennessee, and Mississippi. The only state west of the Mississippi River with a more serious problem in this regard was Nebraska. As mentioned earlier, today the major discrepancy in infant mortality and the major factor in high nonwhite-to-white ratios is the much higher infant mortality among the black population.

In spite of overall substantial improvements in infant mortality rates from the period of the Great Depression

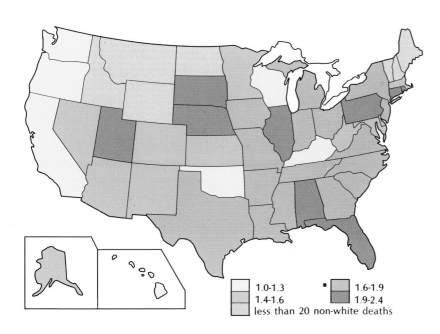

FIGURE 8.8

Infant Mortality: The Number of Non-White Deaths for Every White Death, 1975 (*U. S. average = 1.7)

1.0-1.3   * 1.6-1.9
1.4-1.6   1.9-2.4
less than 20 non-white deaths

FIGURE 8.9

Infant Mortality: The Number of Non-White Deaths for Every White Death, 1985 (*U. S. average = 1.7)

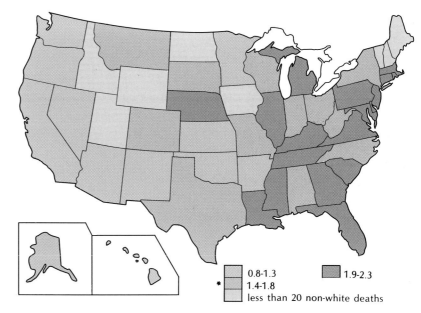

0.8-1.3   1.9-2.3
* 1.4-1.8
less than 20 non-white deaths

to the present, the actual ratio of nonwhite to white infant deaths has changed very little. For example, the national average in 1935 was 1.6 nonwhite deaths for each white infant death. In 1955 the ratio was 1.8:1, and in 1975 and again in 1985 it was 1.7:1. The latest available figures indicate that the ratio of black-to-white infant mortality was about 2.1:1. in 1990. The average infant mortality for white infants was about 8 deaths for every 1,000 live births, whereas for black infants there were approximately 18 deaths. Thus, the mortality rate among black infants was more than twice that among whites. This condition is largely due to socioeconomic differentials between black and white populations.

Urban-Rural Differences

1935. Historically, one of the more important distinctions in the United States with regard to mortality has been the different rates of rural and urban populations. To show the magnitude of infant mortality rate differences between rural and urban areas, the rates for 1935 and 1985 are compared below.

In 1935 the national average infant mortality rate in urban areas was 54 per 1,000 live births, a figure only slightly lower than the 57:1,000 ratio for rural areas (Figures 8.10 and 8.11). In urban areas, infant mortality rates were very high, ranging from 75 to 130 deaths per 1,000 live births among infants born in the

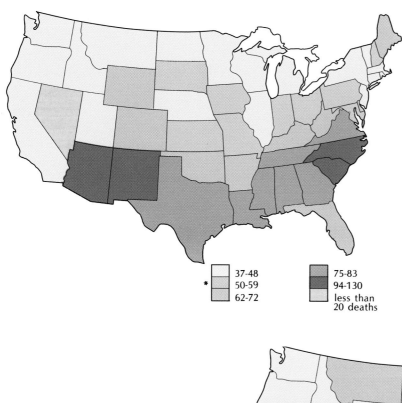

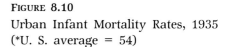

FIGURE 8.10
Urban Infant Mortality Rates, 1935
(*U. S. average = 54)

FIGURE 8.11
Rural Infant Mortality Rates, 1935
(*U. S. average = 57)

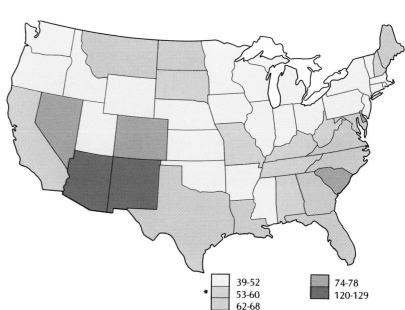

South and the Southwest. In the cities of the Carolinas, New Mexico, and Arizona, extremely high infant mortality ratios of from 94:1,000 to 130:1,000 were reported, at least twice the national average for cities. The lowest rates, from 37 to 48 deaths per 1,000 live births were found in cities of northeastern states such as New York, Massachusetts, and Connecticut, as well as in upper midwestern and far western states.

A somewhat similar pattern may be observed in the geographic distribution of infant mortality rates for children born in rural areas (Figure 8.11) in 1935. With certain exceptions, the highest infant mortality rates, from 74 to 129 deaths per 1,000 live births, were found generally across the southeastern Atlantic Coast states

and especially in the states from Louisiana westward through Nevada. The highest infant mortality rates, from 120 to 129 deaths per 1,000 live births, were found in New Mexico and Arizona. Infant mortality rates in these states were uniformly extremely high in both urban and rural areas. Particularly notable in 1935 in both urban and rural infant mortality rates was the wide range of ratios reported, from 37:1,000 to 130:1,000 in cities and from 39:1,000 to 129:1,000 in rural areas.

1985. By 1985, the urban infant mortality ratio had decreased to a national average of 11.4:1,000 (Figure 8.12) and the rural ratio had decreased to 9.6:1,000

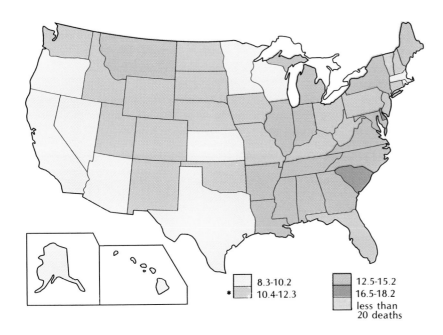

FIGURE 8.12
Urban Infant Mortality Rates, 1985
(*U. S. average = 11.4)

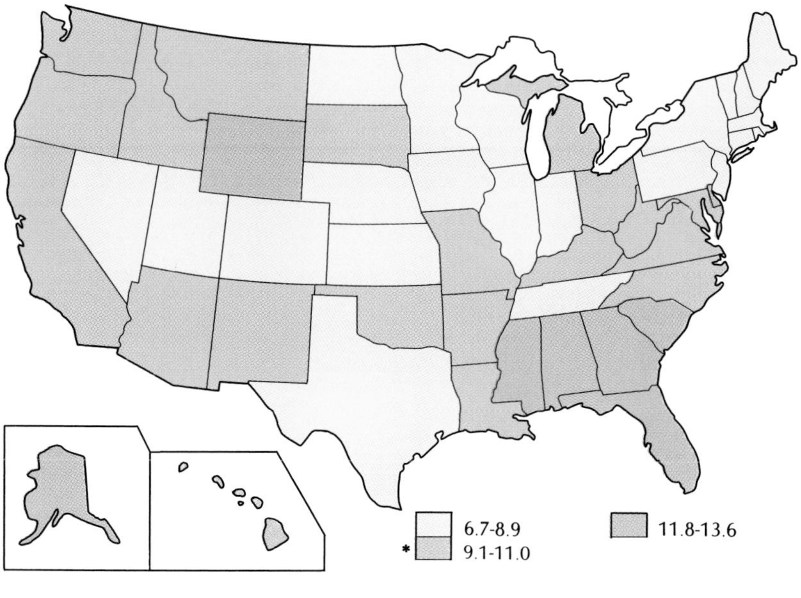

8.3-10.2
* 10.4-12.3
12.5-15.2
16.5-18.2
less than
20 deaths

FIGURE 8.13
Rural Infant Mortality Rates, 1985
(*U. S. average = 9.6)

6.7-8.9
* 9.1-11.0
11.8-13.6

(Figure 8.13). In both urban and rural areas, the largest cluster of high and very high infant death rates occurred throughout most of the southeastern states (Figures 8.12 and 8.13). South Carolina had the highest infant mortality rates in urban areas, up to 18.2 deaths per 1,000 live births. Very high infant mortality ratios, from 12.5:1,000 to 15.2:1,000 were also found in cities of the industrial Midwest, including Michigan and Illinois as well as in New York and Maine in the Northeast.

In rural areas, the lowest infant mortality ratios, ranging from 6.7:1,000 to 8.9:1,000, were regionally concentrated in the northeastern and New England states; across the upper Midwest from Indiana through North Dakota; and in the states across the middle of the country, from Nebraska and Kansas through Nevada. The highest rural infant mortality rates, ranging from 11.8 to 13.6 deaths per 1,000 live births, occurred primarily in states of the Deep South and in Wyoming in the Rocky Mountains. It can be concluded that in these high-infant-mortality states there were extensive pockets of poverty in both rural and urban areas, where the nutritional status of mothers, prenatal care for mothers and children, and neonatal care were insufficient.

Conclusion

A national health objective for the year 2000 is to reduce the infant mortality rate for the total population to fewer than 7 deaths per 1,000 live births. Current efforts are directed toward reducing infant mortality by expanding access to prenatal care for low-income families, as it is believed that prenatal care is likely to have the greatest impact on infant mortality resulting from causes other than birth defects. Program efforts are also emphasizing well-baby care and parenting skills.

Of special interest are attempts to reduce the infant mortality rate among the black population. Historically, the black infant mortality rate has been substantially higher than that of white infants, although the difference has been declining. For example, in 1935 the white infant mortality rate was about 56 and the black rate was about 83 deaths per 1,000 live births. By 1950, the infant mortality rate for whites had declined to 27 deaths per 1,000 live births, while the rate for blacks was about 46. In 1989 the white infant mortality rate was 8.2, in comparison to a black rate of 17.7, more than twice as high as the white rate. The national goal, recognizing this difference, is to reduce the infant mortality rate among blacks to a maximum of 11 deaths per 1,000 live births by the year 2000.

9

AIDS

The presence of acquired immune deficiency syndrome (AIDS) was discovered in the United States in the early 1980s, and by autumn of 1991, almost 200,000 cases of AIDS had been reported in this country alone. Information from the World Health Organization indicates that more than 150 countries around the world are reporting cases of AIDS. Given the advanced state of the disease and the inconsistency of reporting systems in the United States, it is obvious that some U.S. cases are unreported. Assuming further that there are proportionally more unreported cases of AIDS in countries with less developed systems for registering the disease, it can be estimated that there are probably 0.75 million active cases of AIDS in the world today. Compared with the millions of cases of other diseases nationwide and worldwide that existed during the 1980s, the 0.75 million or so AIDS cases do not seem to be particularly significant. Conversely, by the spring of 1992, more than 65 percent of the 210,000 reported cases of AIDS in the United States had resulted in death. Since there is no known cure, it is expected that the remaining 35 percent of people reported to have AIDS will die, as will hundreds of thousands more.

It is quite difficult to forecast the future numbers of AIDS cases that may emerge during the rest of this century. Because of an awareness that there are now many more people who carry the human immunodeficiency virus (HIV) than there are who have already developed the disease AIDS, attention is being drawn to modes of HIV transmission. HIV transmission depends heavily on individual behavior, as well as on social and cultural practices and customs. Specific bio-

logical factors related to individuals and to the virus need to be understood. Short-term projections, from 4 to 5 years, of HIV infection rates and AIDS cases are much more reliable than long-term projections. Current HIV infection rates in the United States range from about 1 million to 1.5 million persons. Some experts claim that there may be between 3 and 4 million persons already affected in North and South America. Worldwide estimates of HIV infection range from 6 to 10 million persons, and some projections to the year 2000 estimate that the number of HIV-infected adults may be as high as 20 million. This means that the total number of AIDS cases is expected to increase substantially during the 1990s. There is therefore a global epidemic or *pandemic* of the disease, and no one has any idea what the final stages of this pandemic may look like. The major reason for this lack of knowledge is that there is neither a vaccine nor a cure for the disease at this time. From a medical standpoint, the pandemic is working its way through the world's population, and there is little the medical and public health communities can do to directly prevent the spread of the disease until either a vaccine or a cure is discovered. The medical community has thus been reduced to a "damage-control" attempt to extend the lives and alleviate the suffering of persons infected with HIV and AIDS.

This situation is particularly unnerving to medical and health care establishments in developing countries. Aside from periodic influenza epidemics, it is generally believed that these nations have undergone an epidemiologic transition wherein increasingly higher mortality rates are attributed to chronic and degenerative diseases such as cancer while lower mortality rates due to infectious diseases are reported each year. In other words, infectious and contagious diseases, which once ranked among the leading killers in developing countries, are now of less consequence. A further result of this circumstance is that the largely chronic diseases, such as heart disease, stroke, and cancer, are becoming more important in some of those countries. Even for these deadly diseases, there are some chances of recovery and cure, to the extent that their numbers can be reduced. This is not true of AIDS.

What then is the health impact of AIDS in the United States and in other developed nations where infectious diseases play a lesser role? Recent improvements in life expectancy for persons with certain AIDS-related diseases have led to suggestions that AIDS might already be "manageable." At the same time, other evidence indicates that life expectancy is decreasing for HIV-infected persons who develop certain aggressive forms of cancer. Also, AIDS victims are vulnerable to a wide range of other illnesses, including tuberculosis (TB). One solution to the problem in developed countries seems to be educational campaigns. In this regard there is some indication, though it is not yet definitive, that educational programs directed toward safer sexual practices in general in the United States have contributed to at least a reduction in the incidence of HIV infection among male homosexuals.

Recently, however, there have been strong indications that the disease is now spreading in a heterosexual pattern among younger population groups. The risk to females is now much greater than it was during the first decade of the epidemic. This finding is particularly important in such locales as Africa, where it is suspected that the disease has been around for a much longer period of time. In many parts of Africa the male-to-female ratio of infected persons is approximately 1:1, and in some age groups there is even some evidence that more females than males have been infected. A similar pattern is emerging in certain Caribbean nations, such as Haiti.

The HIV infection and the AIDS syndrome together constitute a unique and complex phenomenon. Developing an understanding of this phenomenon will require the concentrated cooperative efforts of the medical and the social scientific communities. It is hoped that the ultimate solution will come from medical-biological research and will take the form of vaccines to prevent infection and drugs to rid the body of the virus. Meanwhile, it is imperative for social scientists to concentrate on understanding the virus and its modes of transmission. The social and behavioral contexts of HIV infection and AIDS must be examined. Such an approach should aid in the development of effective programs for controlling the infection process and caring for infected persons.

Etiology and Possible International Origins

It is now known that there is a HIV family. Like other viruses, the HIV is a submicroscopic intercellular parasite. The part of the virus that is important to its survival and spread is ribonucleic acid (RNA), which contains the ingredients necessary to functioning and reproduction. In order to proliferate, the virus extracts necessary ingredients from other cells that are composed of deoxyribonucleic acid (DNA). These agents are part of a group of several retroviruses that are capable of integrating into the chromosome of a host cell and reversing the viral acid into cellular nuclear acid. The retroviruses are also able to copy themselves before returning to the chromosome of a host cell. Retroviruses have properties that are essentially opposite to those of the usual genetic composition, and because the chains of retroviruses are not coated in RNA they must be converted in DNA. In the process, human immune systems are damaged. Specific body sites, or locations, then emerge with infections as the development of the disease AIDS is manifested. With respect to the actual development of AIDS, two human viruses are now known to be involved, HIV-1 and HIV-2. There has been much speculation about the geographic origin of these viruses during the 1980s and the 1990s. Initially, it was thought that HIV-1 was better established than the more recently identified HIV-2; however, some researchers have stated that HIV-2 may have been around longer.

With regard to the origins of the disease, many theories exist. Some of these theories are obviously harder to prove than others. For example, some people believe that HIV is extraterrestrial in origin. Others believe that the viruses were created artificially, either deliberately or by mistake, as part of biological warfare experiments. Another hypothesis links HIV with a strain of swine virus. Still other people believe that it may have been taken back to Europe from the "New World" by the crew of Christopher Columbus, where it lay dormant for centuries. Yet another theory traces HIV to northern European sheep.

While these and other exotic hypotheses have been put forth about the possible origins of HIV, there are three plausible theories about the geographic origin of AIDS, each of which presents difficulties. Only by conducting a search for the origin of the infection and accumulating evidence can its history and geography be more completely elaborated and demonstrated. More important, the search is vital both to development of an understanding of the evolution and transmission of HIV and to development of methods for controlling its biological and social mechanisms. Prevention of AIDS is the real challenge, and understanding the geographical origins of the HIV infection and the mechanisms and geographic dimensions of its transfer may eventually contribute to its control.

To date, the origin of HIV remains a scientific mystery. As with other diseases, such as venereal syphilis, the search for the origins of the HIV will continue for years and we may never know its actual origin with complete assurance. It is important to make the effort, even though the search is not without complications. Throughout much of history, ethnocentricity, inflamed political and social passions, and cultural animosity have led to assignment of blame for the origins of various diseases, especially those which carry the social stigma of association with forms of sexual behavior.

Such was the case during the early phases of the AIDS pandemic. There was a great lack of cooperation by certain nations and the denial of the existence of HIV-related health problems by other countries. An additional complication occurred when early testing procedures for detecting the presence of HIV antibodies in stored serum were found to be imprecise, causing a rather high percentage of false indications of the presence of HIV antibodies. Furthermore, the virus, like many biological organisms, continues to evolve, leading to a periodic redefinition of certain indicator conditions. The clinical expression of infection is incredibly complex as well. There are different types of opportunistic infections and cancers that vary from one population to another and from one geographic area to another.

Despite some of these obstacles, it is possible to identify some general global patterns of infection. The first global pattern occurs largely south of the Sahara in Africa and increasingly in Latin America, especially the Caribbean. In these areas, HIV infection is thought to have begun to spread extensively during the 1970s. Sexual transmission in these largely tropical areas is predominantly heterosexual, and male-to-female ratios of infection are approximately 1:1. In many of these areas the spread of HIV by intravenous drug abusers is relatively rare, but the virus can be spread by repeated use of needles without sterilization and by other common skin-piercing practices.

The second international pattern is found in most of the developed parts of the world, that is, in North America, Western Europe, Australia, New Zealand, and many of the urban parts of Latin America. It seems to be characterized by the spread of HIV during the late 1970s, and most of the early cases occurred among homosexual and bisexual males and intravenous drug abusers.

The third pattern, presently apparent in parts of Eastern Europe, the Middle East, North Africa, and most of Asia and Oceania, and consisting of scattered clusters of AIDS cases and HIV infections, is even more recent in origins. HIV infection appears to have been introduced in these areas during the early to mid 1980s. These countries still account for a small percentage of AIDS cases, but changes have been noted particularly in larger metropolitan areas and in some clusters in Asia where drugs, especially heroin, have been used for long periods of time.

Although no single country or region should be excluded from consideration as the true initial point of origin, these three global patterns suggest that focus on the third pattern would not be useful, but rather that efforts to understand the origins of AIDS should be concentrated on countries that are characterized by the first two patterns. More specifically, international attention has been directed toward selected countries and combinations of regions, namely. Haiti, Euro-America, and equatorial Africa.

The various arrows in Figure 9.1 give some ideas of how the disease might have spread from these three postulated points of origin. The red line shows pathways that might have been followed if HIV had Haitian origins; the purple line shows pathways that might have been followed if the origins were Euro-American; the gray line shows pathways that might have been followed if the early stages of the disease had African origins.

The Haitian Theory of HIV Origin

The idea of Haitian origin offered much ground for speculation during the beginning of the epidemic in the United States. In 1981, practically coinciding with the report of the first cases of AIDS in a male homosexual community in the United States, there were reports of 34 cases of AIDS among Haitian immigrants to the United States as well as 12 previously unrecognized cases in Haiti. The disease was also known, very early in the epidemic, to occur in both men and women in Haiti. What historical possibility might trace the origins of HIV to Haiti through the travels of Christopher Columbus, as mentioned above? It can be conjectured that the crew of Columbus may have taken back to Europe from Hispanola (Haiti) a very contagious and terrifying disease. Traditionally this malady was assumed to have been venereal syphilis.

The more modern Haitian possibility involves the spread of HIV and AIDS or its predecessor to human hosts in Haiti. Since it is possible that the subsequent spread of the epidemic to Western populations, especially in male homosexual communities in the United States, might have taken place in such a fashion, some researchers believe that it originated in Haiti and then spread through international homosexual male tourism. A logical sequence in this theory involves a high level of homosexual contact between Haitians and tourists from North America during the period of so-called gay liberation. Port-au-Prince developed as a regular resort area for homosexual men from the United States. Because of the well-documented high incidence of multiple sexual partners among some homosexual men, it is hypothesized that the infection may have spread very rapidly to tourists and in turn to the tourists' homosexual contacts when they returned to the United States.

It can be further postulated that the infection also traveled from Haiti to central Africa, most notably to Zaire (formerly the Belgian Congo), by way of the migration of a substantial number of middle-class Haitians in the mid-1960s. This travel was a result of the then-recent achievement of independence by Zaire, granted by Belgium. Since the official language of the Belgian Congo had been French, Zaire recruited several thousand French-speaking Haitians to staff the civil service administrative posts left vacant by the departure of the Belgians. Some epidemiologists have assumed that Haitians could have taken the HIV infection to Zaire from their home country. The infection could presumably then have spread across central Africa and into Europe. There are many arguments against this theory of Haitian origin. The one most frequently put forth is that the disease could easily have been imported to Haiti from at least two sources, the United States and Africa.

The Euro-American Theory of HIV Origins

With reference to the Euro-American origin of HIV-related conditions, a large number of reported AIDS cases surfaced in both of these parts of the world almost simultaneously, partly because of the more advanced reporting systems of health conditions among more developed countries. If the hypothesis of germ warfare is disregarded, there appear to be many indications that HIV did not have Euro-American origins. In the early phases of the epidemic, speculation centered on the United States and its male homosexual population. Indeed, the homosexual stamp was affixed to the disease early on, when it was first called "gay-related immunodeficiency (GRID)." In the discussion of the geography of AIDS in the United States, we will present arguments against the idea that the disease originated in the United States.

One biological argument, which was first espoused by researchers who examined the biological similarities between this virus and some viruses found in sheep and goats, is that a version of an animal virus may have mutated into a virus that affects humans. It has also been proposed that HIV is not a new virus—that it has been present among the Euro-American population since the beginning of the twentieth century. Just how a virus might spread to humans from animals poses an even greater problem to researchers than the hypothesis of Euro-American origins. One

possible argument is that a virus closely related to HIV was present in sheep in northern Europe and was somehow transmitted to humans. The virus then lay dormant for many years until it surfaced among homosexuals in the 1970s, and the HIV was then transmitted to Africa in blood and blood products imported from Europe and the United States.

The African Theory of HIV Origin

Retrospective identification of early HIV infection in AIDS cases in some parts of Africa also poses many problems. For example, in many parts of central Africa, clinical record keeping has low priority, and there is a general lack of resources that might permit diagnosis of AIDS by means of technologies used in developed countries. Even amid these problems, and despite continued published claims of a conspiracy among scientists and the media against Africa and Africans, there are some lines of evidence that suggest HIV-1 and the more recently identified HIV-2 had early origins in sub-Saharan Africa. Using more refined and reliable blood tests, some studies, based on a serum sample collected from what was then Leopoldville in the Belgian Congo (now Kinshasa, Zaire), have indicated that HIV-1 may have been present in Africa as early as 1959. In 1970, a pregnant woman in Kinshasa was found to have conditions that would now be considered to be HIV-1 seropositive. In addition, clinical records also indicate a suspected case of AIDS in a Danish surgeon who may have been exposed to HIV-1 in Zaire between 1972 and 1975. There have been many other reports of an AIDS-like illness in central Africa during the late 1960s and the early 1970s. The general term used by Africans for this illness was "slim disease."

Still other evidence indicates the long-standing presence of HIV infection among Africans in remote areas. These groups include Sangaha pygmies and other groups in isolated parts of the Central African Republic. Other examples of early cases of AIDS in Uganda occurred among businessmen who died at an isolated fishing village on Lake Victoria. Although complex and not completely defined, the African origin proposition combines the diffusion of the epidemic on the African continent with a corresponding period of rapid urbanization and international trade. During this period, the migration of young men to cities in search of employment and the development of the infection in prostitutes have especially been documented. Of particular importance in the spread of AIDS is the highway transportation system and specifically the trans-African highway which now links most of the central parts of Africa.

If the initial reservoir of HIV infection was indeed central Africa, the geographic pathways suggested in Figure 9.1 may have accounted for the spread of the

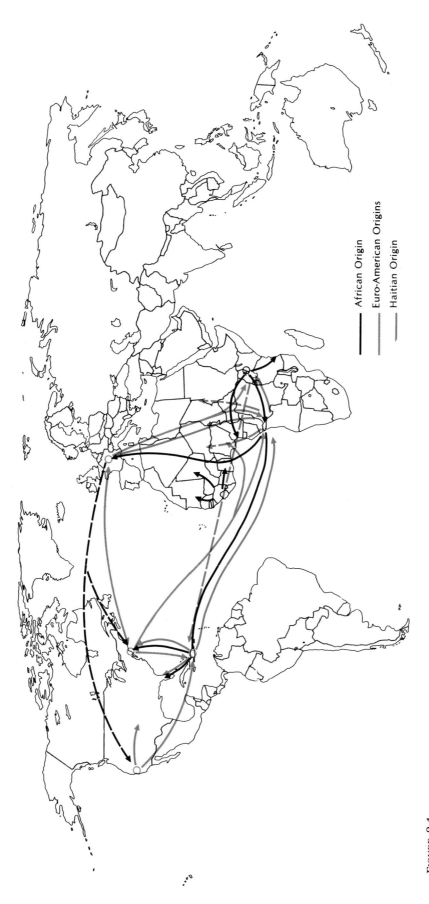

FIGURE 9.1

Three Possible Pathways for the Origin and Diffusion of AIDS

African Origin
Euro-American Origins
Haitian Origin

disease to both Western Europe (because of long-established colonial ties) and America.

However, there are also many difficulties with the African origin theory. One major question that is raised in opposition to this theory is: If Africa is the source of the infection, why was the first clearly defined syndrome identified in American homosexuals and not in Africa? The answer to this question may be related to a lack of appropriate diagnostic facilities in Africa for detecting an emerging syndrome. Then too, early recognition of cases in the United States may have been due to their concentration in limited groups at risk rather than among individuals spread over a larger area such as central Africa.

Which origin theory, if any, is correct? There exists at this time no conclusive scientific evidence that makes it possible to locate the exact geographic origin of HIV. Amid claims and counterclaims, efforts of Western researchers to locate the origins of HIV in Africa have been denounced as a conspiracy and as the perpetuation of racially motivated stereotypes. Furthermore, even within Africa tensions exist in regard to this issue. It is reported that some Nigerian athletes refused to attend the All-Africa games in Nairobi because of the prevalence of AIDS in Nairobi. Certainly, caution must be exercised in interpreting data on HIV infection from any location.

It is, in fact, not known for certain that AIDS is completely a sexually transmitted disease. HIV infection is spread through different types of behavior, and presently the best hope for stopping the epidemic is to change the types of behavior that are responsible for its continued transmission. Yet human behavior and the forces that shape this behavior are among the most complex and poorly understood dimensions of the problem. The knowledge base in the behavioral and social sciences necessary for a search for HIV origins is crude at best. This knowledge is further important in understanding the geography of AIDS as it is now known in the United States.

The Geography of AIDS in the United States

As already indicated, although the specific geographic origins of HIV infection remain unclear at this time, the actual geography of AIDS in the United States can be charted relatively accurately. Information has been made available for a period beginning in 1984 when the Centers for Disease Control started releasing state-based reports of AIDS cases. It can be reasonably argued that, during the 1980s, more public and medical attention in the United States was directed toward HIV and AIDS than toward many other medical conditions.

In addition to the related social patterns of infection and disease, considerable attention was directed toward the geographic aspects of the disease.

The diffusion and distribution of AIDS appear to have followed a standard pattern of spread subsequent to the introduction of HIV within the population. Over a relatively short period of time, HIV infection seems to have filtered from certain large cities to medium-sized centers, then to smaller population centers, and ultimately to suburbs and rural areas. Such a pattern of diffusion is one of several possibilities. However, the geographic spread of HIV is predictable only to a limited extent. Although we acknowledge the lack of hard scientific evidence to support the various origin theories discussed above, it does appear plausible to suggest that HIV infection in the United States was initially introduced primarily through tourism and travel contacts between Haiti and Europe.

Most writers on the geography of the epidemic are in general agreement that the disease appears to have followed an ascertainable sequence of events. For example, the first U.S. cases were probably established during the 1970s, as were the first European cases. Clusters of HIV infections and AIDS cases initially appeared in very specific neighborhoods of certain large cities. Then, outbreaks of AIDS and AIDS-related complexes among homosexual and bisexual males residing in or frequenting certain neighborhoods of New York, San Francisco, Los Angeles, Miami, and Houston began to receive spectacular media coverage. Epidemic reconstruction leads to the conclusion that the HIV epidemic had spread from these urban core nodes more quickly than had been realized, because it was carried by travelers who practiced high-risk behavior. No matter what the specific geographic diffusion pathways may have been, it was well established during the early 1980s that AIDS was a sexually transmitted disease. Eventually, following the city-to-city spread, major core regions and secondary diffusion nodes developed within regions of the country. By the mid-1980s, geographic AIDS corridors could be identified: they were mostly coastal and occurred within densely settled urban areas.

The National Situation

Some AIDS researchers have claimed that the Centers for Disease Control could have released place-specific AIDS reports sooner than 1984. In spite of delays in the release of data on AIDS and AIDS-related complexes, it has been possible to develop a sequence of maps picturing the spread of the disease in the United States during the 1980s. These maps are shown in Figures 9.2 to 9.5. In order to accurately demonstrate the statewide geography of AIDS, given the restrictive characteristics of early at-risk populations, a measure was developed to show the number of cases by state in relation to the relative share of all U.S. AIDS cases. This measure, referred to here as the "AIDS quotient," is derived for each state as follows:

$$\text{AIDS Quotient} = \frac{\text{Percentage of State Population with AIDS}}{\text{Percentage of U.S. Population with AIDS}}$$

By using this measure for a sequence of years, the pattern of AIDS diffusion can be reconstructed. The period 1981–1984, or more specifically, prior to 1984, is shown in Figure 9.2. It is clear that even during the early 1980s, coastal core areas had developed. This pattern follows the theory that AIDS in the United States was of extraneous origin. For example, the early 1980s were characterized by concentrations of reported AIDS cases in New York, California, Florida, Texas, and Colorado. In reality, most of the New York state cases occurred in the New York City metropolitan complex. Similarly, a large share of the California cases occurred in the San Francisco and Los Angeles metropolitan areas. Other early centers of AIDS developed in Denver, Miami, Fort Lauderdale, and Houston.

The net effects of the early downward urban hierarchical diffusion, which probably occurred during the late 1970s, can thus be postulated by examining these maps. By 1984 (Figure 9.3), HIV infection and associated AIDS cases were occurring in relatively large numbers in several of the largest coastal urban areas and in at least one major urban center in the interior of the country. In all likelihood—though these centers were all connected by interstate highways—travel by airline connections was involved in the early diffusion of HIV and the subsequent development of AIDS not only in large metropolitan centers but also in major resort areas. The number and frequency of regular airline flights to and from certain destinations helps to explain the diffusion of AIDS during the early 1980s.

The general pattern which developed in the early 1980s in the United States is probably reflected in the activities of a single individual, a homosexual male airline steward who has been designated "Patient Zero". A significant number of individuals among the first clusters of AIDS cases reported in Los Angeles, San Francisco, and New York were identified as having had sexual relations either with Patient Zero or with other individuals who had previously had sex with him. The emergence of a substantial Gulf Coast pattern is probably associated with the previously described travel of homosexual males from the United States to Haiti, as Patient Zero had done on occasion, and with the migration of infected Haitians to the United States.

The variable yet predominantly slow incubation period of HIV, in contrast to the fast incubation of viruses such as those associated with influenza, means that identification of the probable diffusion pathways of AIDS is comparatively easier than that of some other diseases. For example, Figures 9.6 to 9.7 illustrate the probable diffusion of AIDS beyond the initial parameters of major metropolitan areas. Clearly, secondary patterns of regional spread had developed by the mid-1980s. The expanded national core areas of HIV diffusion at that time were California–Nevada; Colorado; Texas; Florida–Georgia; the northeastern corridor from Boston to Washington, D.C.; and the greater Chicago metropolitan region. By 1986, core areas were thus both coastal and "interior nodal." In other words, there were major concentrations of the disease in specific high-population areas hundreds of miles from the coastal areas. The national pattern of AIDS diffusion in the late 1980s appears to have followed geographic directions which had already been established in previous years and to have been determined by travel on air and highway systems.

By the end of the 1980s, it was possible to identify an AIDS periphery in the United States. For some of the reasons previously mentioned, the infection and associated diseases continue to diffuse both nationally and regionally. The major nodes that had developed during the 1980s had begun to grow together, and by the early 1990s, the AIDS periphery consisted of large parts of the interior western United States as well as many sections that have traditionally been referred to as the "Bible Belt." But even this condition was not permanent. The AIDS periphery collapsed during the late 1980s and the early 1990s.

Regional Aspects of the Spread of AIDS

As the AIDS periphery seemed to grow smaller geographically, and as even more remote rural areas of the United States started reporting increasing numbers of AIDS cases, regional patterns of spread also became more pronounced. The Centers for Disease Control, beginning in 1988, was able to start releasing information on AIDS cases for some large metropolitan areas of the United States—groups of contiguous urban counties referred to as "Metropolitan Statistical Areas" (MSAs). Separating metropolitan AIDS cases from those already reported for states made it possible, by the late 1980s, to identify within-state distributions of AIDS cases to a greater extent than before 1988. This information explains the urban component of AIDS more clearly. For example, in Ohio, the proportions of AIDS cases in metropolitan areas reported by the beginning of 1990 largely coincided with the proportions of the state population residing in the MSAs. That is, the disease had diffused to the point that cases could be predicted on the basis of population distribution.

Regional increases outside metropolitan areas can also be noted for California during the late 1980s.

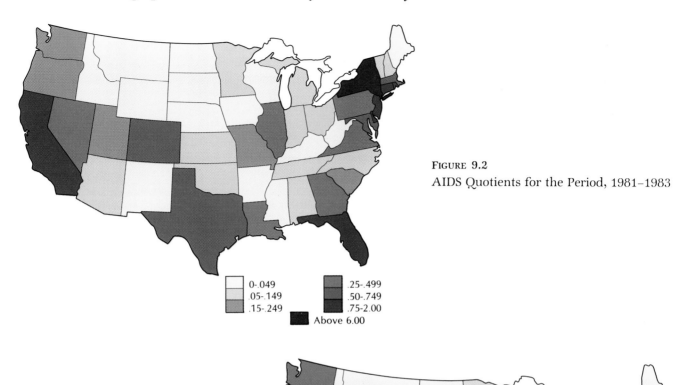

FIGURE 9.2
AIDS Quotients for the Period, 1981–1983

0-.049	.25-.499
.05-.149	.50-.749
.15-.249	.75-2.00
	Above 6.00

FIGURE 9.3
AIDS Quotients for 1984

0-.049	.25-.499
.05-.149	.50-.749
.15-.249	.75-2.00
	Above 6.00

However, in this instance, there were still relatively large numbers of cases of AIDS in the Los Angeles and San Francisco metropolitan areas, two of the original AIDS core nodes. Three cities, San Diego, Anaheim, and Oakland, each contained about 5 percent of the total number of reported AIDS cases in California. Yet, at the beginning of 1990, Los Angeles still accounted for 35 percent and San Francisco for 32 percent of the total number of AIDS cases in the state.

By contrast, a similar comparison of 1990 metropolitan-based data for Florida and Texas showed varying levels of established endemicity. The disease was probably more widespread in Florida than in Texas. For example, the Miami metropolitan area contained

about 30 percent of Florida's AIDS cases, while another 16 percent could be found in the Fort Lauderdale area. These two urban centers were the first to report significant numbers of AIDS cases during the early reporting periods. By 1990, the West Palm Beach and Tampa areas each contained about 11 percent of Florida's cases, while Jacksonville and Orlando each accounted for another 5 percent. In comparison, by the end of the 1980s, Houston remained the center of AIDS in Texas, with 43 percent of the reported cases. Dallas was the other major center, accounting for 24 percent. Other Texas cities with more than 5 percent each included San Antonio (7 percent), Austin (6 percent), and Fort Worth (5 percent).

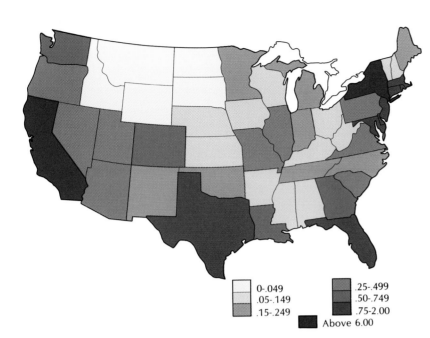

FIGURE 9.4
AIDS Quotients for 1985

0-.049
.05-.149
.15-.249
.25-.499
.50-.749
.75-2.00
Above 6.00

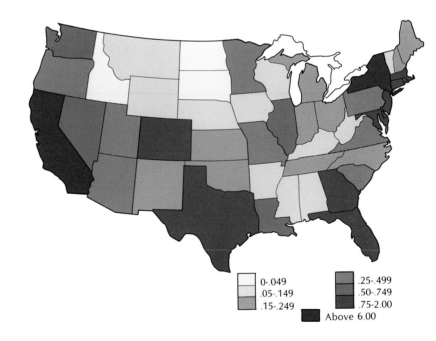

FIGURE 9.5
AIDS Quotients for 1986

0-.049
.05-.149
.15-.249
.25-.499
.50-.749
.75-2.00
Above 6.00

Additional Metropolitan Perspectives on AIDS

The greater New York City area still stands out as the metropolitan area that has had the greatest concentration of reported cases since the onset of AIDS. In spite of the increasing proportions of AIDS cases in other sections of the country, both absolute numbers of AIDS cases and cumulative case rates per 100,000 persons are notable in this area. The cumulative number of AIDS cases in New York City is now about 25,000, which translates into a cumulative case rate approaching 300 per 100,000 people. The rates in adjacent New Jersey are also high, with at least 250 per 100,000 per-

sons in the Jersey City metropolitan area and close to 200 per 100,000 in Newark. In accord with the theory of downward urban filtering, metropolitan rates within the New York region do decline with distance from Manhattan. The Nassau-Suffolk metropolitan area has a rate of about 50 cases per 100,000 persons (near the national average). The Bergen-Passaic metropolitan area has a rate of about 75 cases per 100,000 people. Even Bridgeport, Connecticut, which is farther away but still within the daily commuting field of New York City, has an AIDS rate nearly twice as high as the national average.

In California, declining rates are observed as distance from the San Francisco and Los Angeles nodes of

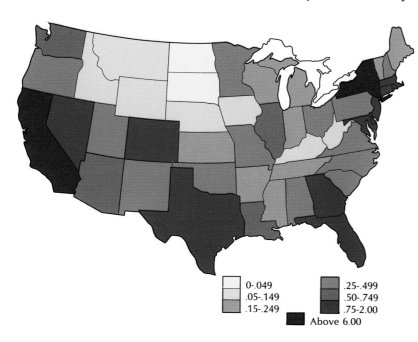

FIGURE 9.6
AIDS Quotients for 1987

0-.049
.05-.149
.15-.249
.25-.499
.50-.749
.75-2.00
Above 6.00

FIGURE 9.7
AIDS Quotients for 1988

0-.049
.05-.149
.15-.249
.25-.499
.50-.749
.75-2.00
Above 6.00

AIDS concentration increases. The San Francisco metropolitan area is approaching a cumulative case rate of close to 500 per 100,000 persons. Across the San Francisco Bay, in Oakland, the rate is about 70 per 100,000. In San Jose, it is only about 35 per 100,000. Thus, the San Francisco AIDS field appears to decline much more steeply than that of either New York or Los Angeles. This decline is due primarily to the presence of a large, geographically concentrated homosexual male community that had shown a rapid course of infection during the early stages of the epidemic.

The Miami metropolitan area, a major early node for the spread of AIDS, has a cumulative AIDS rate of about 175 cases per 100,000 people. To the north,

nearby Fort Lauderdale and West Palm Beach are approaching 150 cases per 100,000 persons. New Orleans, with an AIDS case rate of about 75 per 100,000 persons, has a rate about 1.5 times higher than the national rate but more than 3 times higher than that of nearby Baton Rouge, which has only about 25 cases per 100,000.

The Need for Primary Prevention

The most effective mechanism for dealing with the AIDS problem is primary prevention, which may be achieved by obstructing the spread of AIDS through avoidance of transmission of HIV. While authorities in the field may disagree regarding the amenability of this disease to primary prevention, few would disagree with the need. Not only is treatment costly and sometimes futile, but primary preventive methods can have several desirable spillover effects, including possible reductions in other sexually transmitted diseases, the birth of AIDS-afflicted babies, the use of illicit intravenous drugs, and teenage pregnancy. This is not to imply that primary prevention is simple to achieve, or even that effective methods of achieving it have been found. What it does imply is that primary prevention is important and that ways of stopping the spread of AIDS may have other beneficial societal effects.

10

Alzheimer's Disease

In 1907 a German neuropathologist, Alois Alzheimer (1864–1915) published a short report on the death of a 56-year-old woman who died after an illness which lasted 5 to 6 years. Early symptoms included problems with memory and difficulty in finding her way about, even in her own apartment. At the outset, her motor functions—including strength, coordination, and reflexes—were normal. She died after about 4 years in a mental hospital. Before she died, she had become severely disabled, unable to care for herself, and unable to recognize anyone. Though a similar clinical condition had been accurately described as early as 1838, it was Alzheimer who first accurately described the neuropathology of the disease. He discovered during an autopsy of the woman that she had a high density of brain lesions or plaques on the surface of the brain, the result of degeneration of the tissue. In addition, he described neurofibrillary "tangles" composed of twisted masses of protein. These conditions had been seen previously only in autopsies of brains of people over 70 years of age. For many years this type of finding was considered a medical curiosity and was termed "accelerated aging." Today, the chronic degenerative disease Alzheimer's disease (AD) has been labeled by some researchers "the disease of the century." This dementing illness strips away the aspects of people's lives which are held most precious: the abilities to think; to remember; to interact with loved ones; and to lead productive, happy lives. It should come as no surprise that at the end of the twentieth century AD is one of the most onerous and feared medical disorders.

After a long period of neglect, AD has finally begun to receive considerable scientific scrutiny. Although the cause remains elusive, understanding of the disorder has greatly improved through research. To date there is no way to cure the disease, not even to slow down its progress. Much remains to be learned before progress may be achieved in controlling or eliminating this disorder.

Difficulties in Diagnosis

One of the major problems pertaining to the study of the incidence, pervalence, and epidemiology of AD centers on difficulties in accurate diagnosis. Diagnosis can be made with certainty only through autopsy. A relatively low percentage of people who are believed to have this disease are subjected to autopsy after their death. The major problem in determining the presence or absence of Alzheimer's among the living is difficulty in distinguishing between it and other dementias or behavioral syndromes associated with the general process of aging. These syndromes are generally labeled "senility." Combined clinical and autopsy studies estimate that between 50 and 60 percent of elderly persons with dementia have lesions characteristic of Alzheimer's.

Prevalence

Based on studies of persons 65 years of age and over, it is estimated that there are between 650,000 and

700,000 cases of *severe* AD in the United States. However, to determine the total prevalence, two other groups must be considered: people 65 years of age and over with mild to moderate Alzheimer's and people under 65 years of age with AD. The number of people in the United States in the former group is estimated to be about 300,000 persons. Despite difficulties in determining the prevalence of dementia before age 65, it is likely that between 37,500 and 50,000 Americans under age 60 are afflicted with AD currently.

Combining estimates of all three groups, the current number of cases in the United States is probably about 1 million, at a minimum. This figure represents only part of the story, however, since the continued aging of the population of the United States ensures that the incidence will increase through the remainder of this century and into the next.

The incidence of both senile dementia and AD is increasing. A large part of the increase can be attributed to substantial increases in life expectancy, that is, to the larger percentage of people who have been living longer since 1900. For example, the average life expectancy of persons born in the United States in 1920 was 54 years. For those born in 1950, the life expectancy had increased to over 68 years. By 1991, the average life expectancy had increased to over 75 years, about 72 years for males and over 78 years for females. The increase in life expectancy has moderated in recent years, and relatively slight increases are expected in the future. Particularly important in the recent past, however, was the combination of increased life expectancy with the impacts of the "baby boomers" who were born after the end of World War II in 1945. This large cohort of people will begin to reach age 65 soon after the turn of the century, and many of them can be expected to survive beyond this age due to increased life expectancy. Consequently, large increases in the total number of persons afflicted with Alzheimer's may be anticipated.

It is frequently said, though difficult to document accurately, that Alzheimer's is the fourth or fifth leading cause of death in the United States, after cardiovascular disease, cancer, and cerebrovascular disease. However, the immediate causes of death in patients with senile or presenile dementia of the Alzheimer's type are rather nonspecific. In many cases it is not clear whether or not AD is actually the cause of death. There is no doubt, in any event, that Alzheimer's is a significant health problem, nor that it is increasing as the end of the twentieth century approaches. Yet, as recently as the early 1980s, a standard American textbook of medicine containing over 2,300 pages devoted only 1 page to AD. The National Institute on Aging estimates that over 2 million persons are afflicted with this disease in the United States today, at a yearly cost of over $25 billion and an uncountable cost in social and personal tragedy.

Suspected Risk Factors

As mentioned earlier, no one specific cause or group of causes of AD has been identified. A number of suspected risk factors have been suggested which have been derived from studies of persons with Alzheimer's, their families, and their environments. Among the suggested risk factors are chronological age; genetic inheritance; chromosomal defect (Down's syndrome); advanced parental age; trace elements; transmissible infectious agents, including viruses; immune deficiency or defect; season of birth; and head trauma.

Some studies have found an increased risk of both Alzheimer's and Down's syndrome in blood relatives of patients with onset of AD before age 70. Evidence for the genetic basis of AD has been accumulating for some time. However, though a number of models have been proposed, the precise mode of inheritance is not yet known and may well vary from family to family.

The search for chromosomal correlates of dementia began in the late 1960s. Some researchers have suggested that chromosomal abnormalities or deficits may play a role in Alzheimer's. However, as yet the findings are inconsistent; certainly, they cannot be used to make individual predictions of who is or is not at increased risk of developing the disease.

The Aluminum Hypothesis

A possible role for aluminum as a causative agent or a pathogenic factor in Alzheimer's has at various times been emphasized and debunked. Support for the importance of aluminum comes from studies reporting aluminum deposits as a possible precursor for the development of the neurofibrillary tangles that are characteristic of the disease. Evidence against the aluminum hypothesis derives from lack of development of these tangles in cases of aluminum poisoning and elevations of brain aluminum due to medical conditions. Also, aluminum levels in the cerebrospinal fluid, blood serum, and hair of Alzheimer's patients do not differ from those of the general population. Thus, though existing data do not provide evidence that exposure to high concentrations of aluminum causes AD, they are consistent with the possibility that Alzheimer's patients may be selectively vulnerable to this agent.

The Viral Hypothesis

The possibility that Alzheimer's may be transmitted to humans by an infective agent such as a virus is raised by the similarities of AD to several viral diseases known to be transmissible. While there is some support in favor of a transmissible agent, there is no clinical or epidemiological evidence for human-to-human transmission of the agent, and there is no evidence demonstrating that Alzheimer's patients have a distinctive pattern of infection from conventional viruses.

The Immune System Hypothesis

There is some support for the hypothesis that Alzheimer's is associated with immune system variations. As the immune system begins to deteriorate with age in some persons, there is the increased possibility that environmental toxins that may cause the disease in some persons affect humans to a greater degree.

Head Trauma

A history of head injury with loss of consciousness has been associated with clinically diagnosed AD in several studies. The mechanisms by which single episodes of head trauma could increase the risk of Alzheimer's several decades later are unknown. However, it is known that head trauma with concussion can lead to changes in the blood flow to the brain, leading to exposure to viruses and other toxins, including aluminum.

Conclusion

Presently available data, although they offer interesting clues, do not provide clear scientific support for any particular cause of Alzheimer's. It is possible that some model which has not yet been considered may be the correct one, or that some combination of previously suggested models might explain and predict the occurrence of AD. Alzheimer's may occur because of an interaction between an infectious agent, an environment which causes exposure to the agent, and an individual who may have an inherited or acquired susceptibility to certain agents. It is likely that all three factors play an important role in determining who becomes afflicted with Alzheimer's.

Geographic Patterns in Mortality Rates

Only relatively recently have data become available which estimate the geographic distribution of mortality from Alzheimer's per 100,000 people by state. It is important to use age-adjusted rates when studying AD mortality because of the strong association between the disease and increasing age. Age-adjusted rates eliminate differences between states which may occur because of differences in the age structures of the populations of the states.

1979. In 1979 the national average death rate from Alzheimer's was only 0.4 cases per 100,000 people. In all likelihood this low figure was due to the comparative recency of interest in the disease and in problems related to its definition and clinical diagnosis. Alaska had the highest estimated mortality rate, just 1.1 deaths per 100,000 people (Figure 10.1). Other states with relatively high mortality rates of from 0.5 to 0.9 death per 100,000 people were widely distributed. Of particular interest is the cluster of New England states, including Maine, New Hampshire, Vermont, and Massachusetts, which had very high rates, ranging from 0.7 to 0.9 death per 100,000 people. In the northwest, Washington and Montana had very high mortality rates.

Relatively high mortality rates of from 0.5 to 0.6 deaths per 100,000 people were found widely scattered across the country from Ohio to California and from Wisconsin to Florida.

Extremely low mortality rates of from only 0.05 to 0.10 death per 100,000 population were found in West Virginia, Tennessee, and Mississippi. In fact, Mississippi reported the lowest mortality rate of any state in 1979, fewer than 0.05 death per 100,000 people. Other very low rates of 0.2 death per 100,000 were found in a small cluster of states that included Arkansas, Louisiana, and Oklahoma. Minnesota and Idaho also had low rates in 1979.

1987. As interest in Alzheimer's increased and attempts were made to better clinically define and estimate the number of people who were afflicted with and dying from it, the national average estimated case rate increased dramatically between 1979 and 1987, from 0.4 to 4.2 deaths per 100,000 population. Further, some of the earlier findings pertaining to the geographic distribution of deaths from AD across the nation have been intensified with more recent estimates.

The most recent data which we will cite, those for 1987, are illustrated in Figure 10.2, which shows the distribution of age-adjusted mortality rates for Alzheimer's in 1987. There were an estimated 4.2 deaths from AD for each 100,000 persons in the United States. The age-adjusted rates ranged from a low of 2.1 to a high of 9.2

Very high and high mortality rates from Alzheimer's occurred in both the Northwest and the extreme Northeast. Alzheimer's mortality rates of between 8.6 and 9.2 per 100,000 were found in the western states of Montana and Utah, as well as in New Hampshire, which is located in the extreme Northeast. Montana had the highest mortality rate, 9.2 deaths per 100,000 people, and was closely followed by Utah, with 9.1 deaths per 100,000. Very high rates of from 6.4 to 7.1 deaths per 100,000 people were found in the extreme Northwest, in Washington, Oregon, and Idaho, as well as in Maine and Vermont in the extreme Northeast.

States with high mortality rates from Alzheimer's, ranging from 5.2 to 6.1 deaths per 100,000 population, included Wyoming, Colorado, Arizona, and Nevada in the West. In the East, high rates were found in the coastal states, including Massachusetts, Virginia, North Carolina, and Georgia.

Thus, in 1987 there were two significant geographic clusters of states with high to extremely high mortality rates from AD. One of these clusters occurred in the extreme northeastern New England states, from Massachusetts through Maine. The largest geographic cluster of states with these high rates occurred in the western portion of the country, however. With the exception of California and New Mexico, all the states in the western one-third of the country had higher mortality rates than the national average.

At the other end of the spectrum, there were two small clusters of states with extremely low mortality rates due to Alzheimer's, that is, from 2.1 to 3.5 deaths per 100,000 population. Interestingly, one of these clusters was adjacent to the New England cluster of states that had very high and extremely high mortality rates. The northeastern states of New York, Pennsylvania, and New Jersey had mortality rates ranging from 2.1 to 3.5 deaths per 100,000 people. New York had the lowest mortality rate in the country, only 2.1 deaths from Alzheimer's for every 100,000 persons. In the southern states along the Mississippi River, including Arkansas, Mississippi, and Louisiana, there was another cluster of states with very low mortality rates, 3.4 per 100,000 in each. Michigan with 2.9 deaths per 100,000, North Dakota with 3.1, and Alaska with 2.7 were the other states which fell into this very low category.

Generally, states in the midsection of the United States, from West Virginia westward to Nebraska, and from Minnesota southward to Texas, had average to lower-than-average mortality rates due to Alzheimer's.

The 1987 geographic pattern of deaths from Alzheimer's disease is both interesting and puzzling. The 1979 pattern of states with both low and high mortality rates has been intensified by the more recent data. On the one hand, there certainly appear to be some important and significant emerging clusters of states with very high to extremely high AD mortality rates. This clustering occurs most notably in the western half of the United States and, to a lesser extent, through much of New England. At the same time, extreme diversity in the climates, urban populations, and population characteristics of these states must be noted. Similar diversity occurs in the small clusters of states with extremely low case rates in the Northeast and along the Mississippi River in the South.

Changes in Mortality Rates

1979–1987. In the period 1979–1987, Alzheimer's was listed as the underlying cause of death for over 46,000 people. The national average mortality rate from AD increased from 0.4 to 4.2, an increase of 3.8 deaths for each 100,000 persons. The 1987 rate was almost 10 times as high as the 1979 rate. The greatest increase in the death rate occurred among people 80 years of age and over. In 1979 the death rate from Alzheimer's in this group was 3.8 per 100,000 persons; by 1987, this rate was 108.8 per 100,000. For persons between 70 and 79 years of age, the death rate increased from 2.7 deaths per 100,000 persons in 1979 to 28.4 per 100,000 in 1987. Increases in death rates in younger age groups were much lower. Rather than representing actual increases in death rates, the observed increases are probably due primarily to increased sensitivity to and recognition of death resulting from Alzheimer's and related causes.

Geographic changes in mortality rates related to Alzheimer's between 1979 and 1987 are illustrated in Figure 10.3. During this period every state experienced an increase in this mortality rate. The largest increases appear to have occurred primarily in states with relatively high mortality rates in 1979. Thus, with certain exceptions, the map depicting increases in mortality rates between 1979 and 1987 very closely resembles the map of 1987 mortality rates. For example, the largest increases took place in the western states and in New England—by and large the same clusters of states that had the highest mortality rates in 1987. For example, in the period 1979–1987, Montana, Utah, and New Hampshire had mortality rate increases of 8.5, 8.6, and 7.9 deaths per 100,000 population, respectively. Furthermore, in 1987 these states also had the highest mortality rates. Similarly, in the same period, states such as Washington, Oregon, and Idaho had very high mortality rate increases, from 5.8 to 6.7 per 100,000 people. The mortality rates in these states also ranked among the highest in 1987.

Very low increases in mortality rates from AD occurred in states such as New York (which had an increase of 1.8 deaths per 100,000 population), Pennsylvania (2.7 per 100,000), New Jersey (3.1 per 100,000), Michigan (2.6 per 100,000), and North Dakota (2.8 per 100,000). In 1987 these were among the states with the lowest Alzheimer's mortality rates. Though states such as Louisiana, Mississippi, and Alabama had relatively modest increases of from 3.2 to 3.7 deaths per 100,000 people between 1979 and 1987, their mortality rates were among the lowest in 1987. Finally, while Alaska had an extremely high mortality rate in 1979, its death rate increase was the lowest in the period 1979–1987—an increase of only 1.6 deaths per 100,000. As a

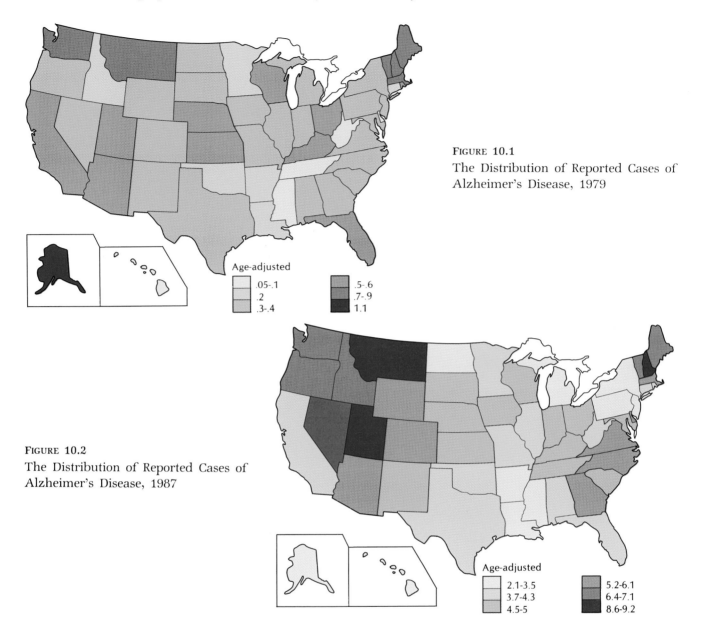

FIGURE 10.1
The Distribution of Reported Cases of
Alzheimer's Disease, 1979

FIGURE 10.2
The Distribution of Reported Cases of
Alzheimer's Disease, 1987

result, in 1987 Alaska had one of the lowest Alzheimer's mortality rates in the nation.

Because of relatively few autopsies which are performed and because of the difficulty in clinically diagnosing Alzheimer's among the living, care must be used in assessing the reported mortality rates. At the same time, using standard criteria and estimating procedures, significant changes in mortality rates are apparent in the period 1979–1987. Moreover, the distribution of these changes has resulted in an intensification of the geographic clusters of both very high and

very low mortality rates across the nation. It is important to monitor these changes and their distribution. Although to date it is very unclear what factor or factors are responsible for AD, current hypotheses pertaining either to factors in the environment (such as aluminum) or to genetic differences in the population might be supported by further geographic assessment of death rates. Alternatively, the geographic patterns may suggest other hypotheses to be studied in the search for the cause of this increasingly prevalent disease.

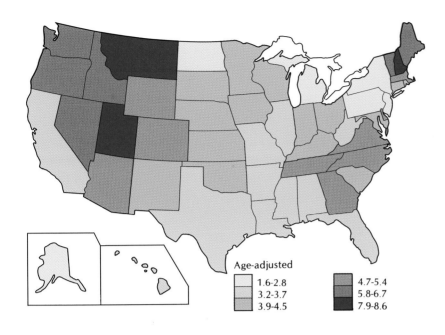

FIGURE 10.3
The Difference in Reporting of
Alzheimer's Disease, 1979–1987

11

Motor Vehicle Fatalities

Development of the Automobile Industry

Like the motor vehicle itself, the automotive industry originated in Europe. The commercial manufacture of automobiles began in France and Germany about 1890. Britain also had some early pioneers in automobile development. Interestingly, however, British progress was generally impeded by the passing of the so-called red flag law in 1865, which required that self-propelled vehicles on public highways be preceded by a man on foot carrying a red flag. It was only after the repeal of this law in 1896 that the British automotive industry developed.

Except for about a dozen cars produced by Charles Edgar Duryea and his brother J. Frank Duryea, in Springfield, Massachusetts, between 1893 and 1898, commercial production of automobiles in the United States began in 1897 with the Pope Manufacturing company of Hartford, Connecticut, and the Winton Motor Carriage Company of Cleveland, Ohio. The Olds Motor Vehicle Co. (1898) quickly followed and then came Packard (established in 1900), Cadillac (1900), Buick (1900), Ford (1903), and Maxwell-Briscoe (1903). Henry Ford had two false starts before he founded the Ford Motor Company in 1903 with a $28,000 loan from a group of Detroit businessmen.

Few technical innovations have received as enthusiastic a reception as the motor vehicle. The demand for automobiles was so great that the fledgling industry of the 1890s became big business during the following

decade. In 1900 a total of 4,192 passenger cars were sold in the United States. This figure increased to 181,000 in 1910 and to 1,905,000 by 1920. Some 2,900 different U.S. automobile-producing firms appeared before World War I. To meet the demand for automobiles, Henry Ford introduced the moving assembly line in 1913 in a new factory located in Highland Park, Michigan. In 1921 the Ford Motor Company was moved to the massive River Rouge plant in Dearborn, Michigan. Some 15 million Model T Ford automobiles were manufactured and assembled before this type of automobile was discontinued in 1927.

The automobile industry did not escape the world-wide depression of the 1930s. Production dropped from a peak of 5 million vehicles in 1929 to a low of just over 1 million in 1932. Output was to climb rather steadily thereafter; however, the 1929 figure was not exceeded until some 20 years later.

When World War II began, Ford was one of the leading automobile manufacturers. The other two were its competitors Chrysler and General Motors. All three of these leading companies converted from building automobiles to aiding the war effort. After the war, automotive production had to be significantly increased to match the demand. In 1940 about 3,700,000 passenger cars were sold in the United States. By 1950, the sales had more than doubled, to 6,700,000. Since that time, annual sales of passenger cars have varied between 5 million and 8 million.

In the twentieth century the automobile emerged as the dominant innovation which was to change the fabric of U.S. society. Today the country is dominated by the culture of the automobile. In 1903 the first recorded transcontinental trip by automobile was recorded. In 1990 approximately 2 trillion vehicle-miles of travel were completed by drivers in the United States. Despite increasing problems related to automobile pollution and decreasing fuel resources necessary to run them, Americans' penchant for the automobile and the freedom of travel it permits continues to flourish.

What frequently seems to be ignored, however, is the large number of deaths annually attributed to motor vehicle accidents. Today, these crashes are the leading cause of death in the United States among persons aged 1 to 34. In addition, 40 percent of all motor vehicle-related deaths occur among persons aged 15 to 24. Perhaps Americans have become inured to the bloodshed on U.S. streets and highways. Every day, almost every newspaper in the country publishes reports of people dying in automobile accidents. To put it in perspective, it is estimated that more than 500,000 people died in automobile accidents in the period 1980–1990, whereas battle deaths in all the wars in which American forces have participated have totaled approximately 578,000. In other words, approximately as many Americans died on U.S. highways in 10 years as in *all* wars in American history, from the Revolutionary War through the Persian Gulf war.

Mortality Rates

Per 100,000 Population

In 1906, the first year for which data are available, the average national mortality rate from motor vehicle accidents was 0.5 death per 100,000 persons. There was an increase in mortality rates each year through 1931 (Figure 11.1). By 1931 the mortality rate had risen to

27.2 deaths for every 100,000 residents of the United States. It has become apparent that travel decreases during times of economic recession or depression, and this decrease is associated with a decrease in mortality rates. Thus, in 1932, during the depths of the Great Depression, the mortality rate declined to 23.6 deaths per 100,000 persons. The mortality rates began to climb subsequently, increasing to 30.8 per 100,000 persons in 1937. The rates decreased during the next 3 years but jumped up again, rising to 30 deaths per 100,000 persons in 1940. The influence of World War II, including the reduced availability of new cars, gas rationing, and the absence from the nation's highways of hundreds of thousands of men who were serving overseas, is reflected in a sharp downward shift in the mortality rates from motor vehicle accidents. In the period 1941–1942, the mortality rate decreased from 30 to about 21 deaths for every 100,000 people. In 1943 the death rate declined to 17.8 deaths per 100,000 people, the lowest since 1924; this 1943 rate continues to hold the record for the lowest rate since 1924. The death rate began to rise as the war wound down; it fluctuated between 21 and 24 deaths per 100,000 over the next decade. In times of recession, such as 1960–1961, the death rate again decreased.

By 1973 the death rate had risen to 26.3 per 100,000 persons. In 1974, however, the death rate obviously decreased substantially, to 21.8 deaths per 100,000. This period was influenced by the oil crisis, which was characterized by long lines at gas pumps, significant increases in the cost of gasoline, and the imposition of a nationwide highway speed limit of 55 miles per hour. These factors and the recession that occurred at the same time combined to have a significant impact on the mortality rate from motor vehicle accidents. Over the past several years the national average mortality rate from motor vehicle accidents has stabilized at about 20 deaths for every 100,000 persons. Accord-

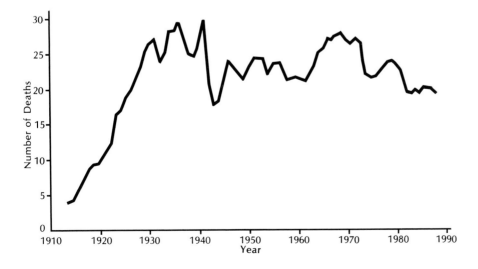

FIGURE 11.1
Motor Vehicle Fatalities: Deaths per 100,000 Persons

ing to the most recent data available, in 1988 the death rate from motor vehicle accidents was 19 for every 100,000 persons in the United States.

Per 100 Million Vehicle-Miles

Since about 1923, it has been possible to compute the average annual mortality rate from motor vehicle accidents per 100 million vehicle-miles (Figure 11.2). In 1923, an estimated 85 million vehicle-miles were traveled by all motor vehicles in the United States. While this seems a rather large number, it pales in comparison with the current estimates of over 2 trillion vehicle-miles traveled in this country annually. From a rate of 21.7 fatalities per 100 million vehicle-miles in 1923, the average annual rate has declined to about 2.3 fatalities per 100 million vehicle-miles in 1988.

This figure certainly reflects a substantial improvement, probably the result of better-engineered automobiles and better highway construction, as well as stricter law enforcement and advances in passenger safety features. However, the average annual number of motor vehicle deaths has increased from 6,700 in the post-World War I period to more than 47,000 in 1988. The 1988 figure reflects a slight reduction in the annual number of deaths over several years. Since 1962 the annual number of deaths resulting from automobile accidents has been greater than 40,000, and from 1966 through 1983, it exceeded 50,000—almost 55,000 in 1970, for example, and 54,000 in 1981. Thus, over the past 20 years, approximately 1 million or more persons have died in motor vehicle accidents. This is a tragic figure and a high price to pay for increased mobility. There are additional risks to health from motor vehicle-caused air pollution.

Geographic Patterns in Mortality Rates

Per 100,000 Persons

1935. In 1935 the average number of deaths from motor vehicle accidents was 27 per 100,000 population. As illustrated in Figure 11.3, the lowest mortality rates from automobile accidents occurred in a belt of states extending from the upper Midwest, including Minnesota and North Dakota, southward to Louisiana, Mississippi, and Alabama on the Gulf of Mexico. Another area with low mortality rates occurred the upper Northeast; these states included Maine, New Hampshire, Connecticut, New York, and Pennsylvania. High mortality rates, ranging from 37 to 51 deaths per 100,000, occurred principally in southwestern states such as California, Arizona, and New Mexico. Other states with the highest mortality rates included Wyoming and Florida. Nevada, with a mortality rate from automobile accidents of 78 per 100,000 people, stood out as the highest in the nation.

1950. Deaths from automobile mortality during the 1950s averaged about 24 to 25 per 100,000. Regional variations within the United States for 1950 are depicted within Figure 11.4. The most important aspect of change in automobile death patterns from 1935 to 1950 is that during that time period, the role of the automobile in U.S. society had changed drastically. During the Great Depression of the 1930s, the automobile was still being used by many for recreation instead of a major mode of journey-to-work transportation. Also, not nearly so many Americans had cars in the 1930s as in the 1950s. The post-World War II era was characterized by a boom in automobile production due to increasing demand and the ability to pay for newer,

FIGURE 11.2
Motor Vehicle Fatalities: Deaths per 100,000,000 Miles

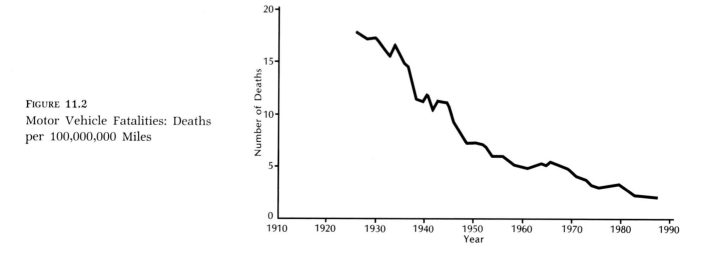

bigger, and faster cars. Perhaps the most striking change in geographical variations in the national pattern of deaths caused by automobiles consisted of extremely high rates in the western part of the country. For example, Wyoming, Idaho, Nevada, Arizona, and New Mexico all reported rates from one and one-half to two times the national average. These states all contain vast areas of open roads as well as many mountains. In addition, Oregon, California, Montana, Utah, Colorado, South Dakota, Kansas, and Texas all reported above-average rates. These states also contained long stretches of highways with limited adjacent development during the 1950s, and most of the roads were two-lane then. Another regional cluster of higher than average automobile deaths that had developed by 1950 was in the Southeast. This region is the home of stock car racing, and many claim this tradition is partially related to an automobile culture that evolved in that region. Even today, many Southeastern states have some of the highest ratios of automobile parts establishments per capita in the United States. The states that ranked average for automobile deaths in 1950 included many in the Ohio and Mississippi Valley Regions: Minnesota, Wisconsin, Iowa, Nebraska, Illinois, Missouri, Oklahoma, Arkansas, Louisiana, Kentucky, Tennessee, Ohio, and West Virginia. Higher than average rates for Michigan and Indiana can be attributed to general proximity to Detroit and higher than average automobile ownership and use in 1950. The Northeast reported lower than average death rates in 1950. This phenomenon can be attributed to greater use of public transportation in that part of the U.S. in 1950. Lower than average rates for Mississippi and North Dakota in 1950 were no doubt due to lower levels of automobile ownership in poor areas of the rural south and Native American reservations in the Dakotas.

1970. By 1970, the national average mortality rate from automobile accidents had declined to 23 deaths per 100,000 people. States with much lower than average mortality rates were clustered in the highly urbanized northeastern section of the United States (Figure 11.5). Nine of the ten states with mortality rates ranging from 11 to 19 deaths per 100,000 people were located in the Northeast. Only North Dakota provided an exception to this pattern. States with about average rates, ranging from 20 to 25.8 deaths per 100,000, were again found in a belt stretching from the upper Midwest to the Gulf of Mexico, but by this time, Ohio, West Virginia, and Virginia were included. The highest mortality rates, ranging from 37 to 51 deaths per 100,000, occurred in some of the least densely populated states in the West, including Idaho, Wyoming, Nevada, Arizona, and New Mexico.

1988. By 1988, the national average of deaths resulting from motor vehicle accidents had decreased to 19 deaths per 100,000 persons (Figure 11.6). Again, consistently with past geographic patterns, the most densely settled states of the northeastern United States had rates among the lowest in the nation, ranging from 13 to 17 deaths per 100,000 persons. Added to this group in 1988 were states in the upper and central Midwest, including North Dakota, Minnesota, and Wisconsin as well as Nebraska and Colorado.

Two clusters of states stood out in 1988 with very high motor vehicle mortality rates per 100,000 population. These were in the Southeast (South Carolina, Georgia, and Florida) and in the Southwest (New Mexico, Arizona, and Nevada). In these states, as well as in Wyoming, the motor vehicle fatality rates ranged from 32 to 38 deaths per 100,000 persons.

Per 100 Million Vehicle-Miles

When comparing automobile deaths per 100 million vehicle miles and per 10,000 automobiles, overall trends this century generally decrease with time (Figures 11.2 and 11.7). These decreases can be attributed in more recent years to better highway design and construction, federally-mandated safety improvements in automobile construction, and an increasing awareness of deaths attributed to alcohol consumption. While trends generally leveled off during the 1980s and early 1990s due to decreased speed limits over the previous two decades, many years of improvements in high school driver education courses have definitely had a positive effect. As mentioned below, automobile death rates in general can be lowered even more through stronger drunk-driving laws and alcohol awareness programs.

1970. In 1970 the national average death rate from motor vehicles was 4.8 deaths per 100 million vehicle-miles (Figure 11.8). What might be termed "average" death rates, from 3.8 to 6.0 deaths per 100 million vehicle-miles, were distributed across the country from Maine to the Northwest and from the Dakotas to Texas. Particularly notable, however, were the clusters of states in the Southeast and in the Rocky Mountains and southwestern areas. A solid core of states with very high death rates from motor vehicles, 6.1 to 7.6 deaths per 100 million vehicle-miles, was located in the Southeast. From Tennessee to Louisiana to South Carolina, very high mortality rates occurred. In the West, from Montana and Idaho southward to Arizona and New Mexico, very high mortality rates from vehicle accidents were also reported.

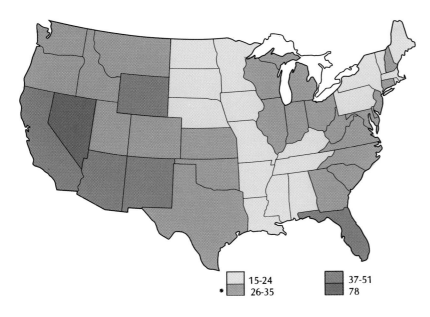

Figure 11.4

Motor Vehicle Fatalities per 100,000
Persons, 1950 (*U. S. average = 23)

1988. By 1988, the pattern had become quite irregular (Figure 11.9). The greatest change appeared to be an improvement in some of the southeastern states: Tennessee, Alabama, Louisiana, and Georgia. In 1988 these states had mortality rates ranging from 2.5 to 2.9, as compared to the national average of 2.3 deaths per 100 million vehicle-miles. Wyoming and Arizona in the West, as well as Alaska in the North, had improved their mortality rates. Remaining in the very high category, with rates from 3.2 to 3.3 deaths per 100 million vehicle-miles, were West Virginia, South Carolina, and Mississippi in the Southeast and Idaho, Nevada, and New Mexico in the West. Relatively low mortality rates, from 1.7 to 2.0 per 100 million vehicle-miles were distributed from Vermont and Connecticut

in the Northeast across North Dakota, Minnesota, and Wisconsin in the upper Midwest to Washington in the Northwest.

Conclusion

Annual death rates from motor vehicle crash injuries per 100,000 U.S. residents decreased 10 percent between 1940 and 1980. However, this small change masked increases in motor vehicle crash death rates among young adults and major decreases in the rates among the elderly. Regardless of the exact causes, there was an 84 percent increase in the number of years of life lost in motor vehicle crashes before age 70.

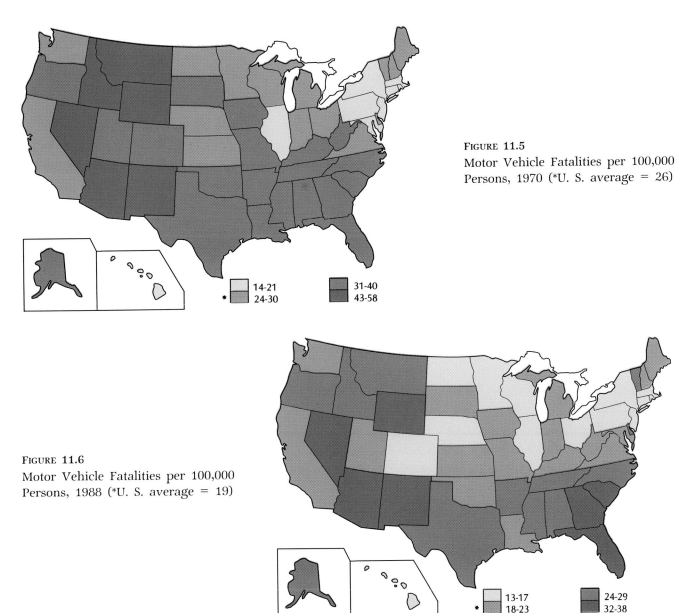

FIGURE 11.5
Motor Vehicle Fatalities per 100,000 Persons, 1970 (*U. S. average = 26)

FIGURE 11.6
Motor Vehicle Fatalities per 100,000 Persons, 1988 (*U. S. average = 19)

To the extent that these changes in mortality patterns were reflected in morbidity, it is reasonable to predict future increases in the numbers of young persons who will be chronically disabled by motor vehicle crash injuries.

Among the principal factors contributing to very high death rates among young people is alcohol consumption, which is involved in about 50 percent of fatal crashes. A recent study estimated that eliminating alcohol consumption by drivers would reduce traffic fatalities from 42 to 51 percent. The magnitude of this potential reduction suggests that intervention to reduce drunk driving would be very valuable.

State-by-state mapping of death rates has revealed major regional variations. High motor vehicle-related death rates in western states have at times been attributed to the greater distances driven in those states. Even when data are adjusted for amount of travel, however, rural areas still have high rates. Poor roads may play a major contributing role in raising death rates in areas of low population density. Several studies have found that the highest death rates occurred in the western half of the United States and in counties with the lowest populations per square mile. A road's gradient and width and the presence or absence of adequate shoulders and guardrails all contribute to the increased probability and severity of crashes. Other factors thought to contribute to this pattern include differences in road characteristics, travel speeds, types of vehicles, and available trauma services. Especially low

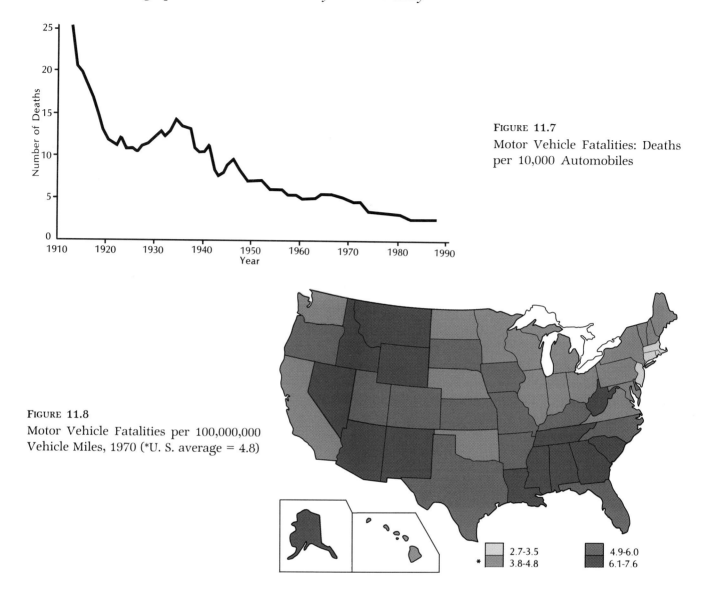

FIGURE 11.7
Motor Vehicle Fatalities: Deaths per 10,000 Automobiles

FIGURE 11.8

Motor Vehicle Fatalities per 100,000,000 Vehicle Miles, 1970 (*U. S. average = 4.8)

2.7-3.5	4.9-6.0
* 3.8-4.8	6.1-7.6

injury rates in a state or region may also suggest protective factors such as the elimination or relocation of utility poles, strict law enforcement pertaining to drunk or other drug-impaired driving, and mandatory driver education. Unless and until the problem is addressed directly and effectively, the nation will continue to lose thousands of lives needlessly each year through motor vehicle accidents.

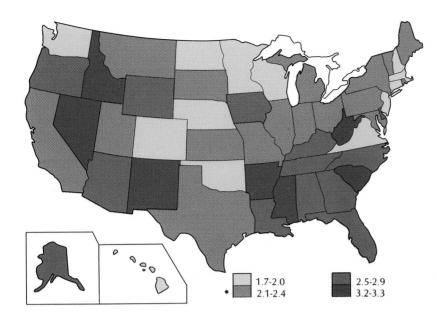

FIGURE 11.9
Motor Vehicle Fatalities per 100,000,000
Vehicle Miles, 1988 (*U. S. average = 2.3)

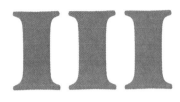

Medical Care
Resources and
Treatment Facilities

12

Physician Supply and Distribution

If provision of medical care were simple and straightforward, there would be little need for discussion of *physician demography*: the supply and distribution of physicians. Because it is complex, however, reaching agreement about how many doctors (let alone considerations of what types of doctors) a community needs is difficult or impossible. There are even problems associated with attempts to define "community" in a way that would be appropriate to the measurement of physician distribution. Finally, there is the problem of lack of evidence directly linking the number of doctors in a community to the health status of its residents. Many factors pertaining to the health of any individual and of the community as a whole lie beyond the realm of physician intervention and are more closely related to individual behavior and organized public health measures.

Nevertheless, physicians continue to be the keystone of the health enterprise and medical care experience of most people in the United States. The vast majority of people turn to a physician for care and comfort when they are faced with acute and chronic medical conditions, from minor ailments to the life-threatening sicknesses. Physicians will remain central to the medical care process in the foreseeable future, and it is therefore appropriate for us to discuss the evolution of physician demography in the United States in the twentieth century.

Nineteenth-Century Concerns

The number of physicians practicing in each state and some measure of their quality were important matters to delegates to the first National Medical Convention in 1847. Delegates were instructed to determine as far as was practicable the numbers of men who were practicing medicine in their respective states. This was apparently the first U.S. attempt to systematically collect information on the number of physicians in each state. In 1850 the U.S. Census reported a total of 40,564 practicing physicians—a physicians-to-population ratio of about 175:100,000, or 1 physician for each 571 people.

There is also evidence of early concern about replacing and replenishing the supply of physicians. In the mid-1850s, an attempt was made to predict an expected "vacancy" rate of physicians per year to be filled by medical school graduates. The number of practicing physicians increased to 50,000 by the end of 1870. In 1870, therefore, there were 128 physicians for every 100,000 people in the United States. By 1895, there were 200 physicians for every 100,000 people residing in the United States—64 percent higher than the ratio (128:100,000) 25 years earlier. Many of these physicians were perceived to be matriculating through less than adequate medical schools, however.

Concern was also expressed about the possibility that the United States had excessive numbers of doctors and medical schools for the population. Concern was directed especially at the proliferation of inadequate medical schools and the lack of well-educated physicians being turned loose upon communities. It was believed then, as now, that a good doctor is much better than a poor doctor but only little better than no doctor. Some people thought that a poorly educated physician might do more harm to patients than leaving them untreated.

Review and Reform in the Twentieth Century

Concern about inadequate medical training led to two major reviews of medical education in the United States shortly after the turn of the century. In 1905 the Council on Medical Education noted five states with weak programs in medical education: Illinois, Kentucky, Maryland, Missouri, and Tennessee. While this report was important, the report entitled *Medical Education in the United States and Canada*—the so-called Flexner Report, which was written by Simon Flexner and published in 1910—had a more far-reaching effect on medical education and the production of physicians in the United States. This strongly worded report concluded that the country was suffering from an excess of underqualified physicians. The author believed this to be the result of a century of over-production of doctors which resulted in too many physicians, with even the smallest towns being oversupplied with low-grade practitioners. Towns with total populations of fewer than 100 persons had as many as 5 physicians, and towns with fewer than 50 residents frequently had 2 or more.

While few states and sections of the country emerged unscathed in this report, special criticism was directed at southern medical schools. The South was considered to be generally overcrowded with substandard medical schools with which nothing could be done. For example, in Alabama satisfactory medical education could not be found. In Arkansas neither of two medical schools had a very good evaluation. The outlook in Kentucky was not promising and the University of Louisville was singled out as without resources and the University of Kentucky was totally unequal to the task of providing medical education because it was judged to have low standards. Indeed, Kentucky was delineated as one of the largest producers of low-grade doctors in the country.

Though the South suffered severe criticism as a region, states in other areas also received barbed and stinging criticisms. For example, Oregon's two medical schools were considered to be without resources and ideals. The Flexner Report said that there was no justi-

fication for their existence, the state will do well to eliminate them. Chicago did not fare any better in the Flexner Report.

The report called for development of medical education based on the German model of a university function, thus denying any role for proprietary schools. Further, it called for a drastic reduction in the number of medical schools in the nation, from the existing 155 to 31. Each would provide a 4-year curriculum and be limited to no more than 70 graduates per year. Such recommendations, of course, affected the lives of many. Simon Flexner's life was reportedly threatened. Libel suits were considered, and some were even brought to court.

The impact of the Flexner Report, higher state board requirements for practice, and the financial difficulties of many proprietary medical schools drastically reduced the number of practicing physicians and the production of physicians in the United States. Between 1904 and 1915, an estimated 92 medical schools merged or closed their doors. The number of medical schools in the nation was 95 in 1915 and only 85 in 1920. Whereas in 1906 the 162 medical schools had been producing over 5,300 physicians annually, in 1920 the 85 schools were training just over 3,000 physicians per year. In 1910 the "physician density" in the United States was about 157:100,000. It fell to 142 in 1916 and further declined to 126:100,000 in 1931.

Geographic Patterns of Physician Distribution

1906–1933. In 1906 there were an estimated 120,000 physicians in the United States and a national average of 152 physicians per 100,000 population. The ratios ranged from 73:100,000 in South Carolina to 360:100,000 in Montana. South Carolina and North Carolina (with 74:100,000) had the lowest physicians-to-population ratios in 1906. Two regions of the United States, the South and the upper Midwest, were characterized by rather low physicians-to-population ratios (Figure 12.1). Ratios from Louisiana eastward to Florida were between 101:100,000 and 123:100,000, a range which was also found in the Dakotas, Minnesota, and Wisconsin. In the same category, the lowest ratios were generally found in the South. Only Georgia (with 119:100,000) had more than 110 physicians per 100,000 population. Conversely, only Minnesota (with 105:100,000) among the northern states had fewer than 110 physicians per 100,000.

About average (152:100,000) physicians-to-population ratios, ranging from 138:100,000 to 162:100,000, were found throughout the northeastern states from Maine southward; through West Virginia; in the central midwestern states of Iowa, Nebraska, and Kansas; and in Oregon and Idaho in the far West. A cluster of moderately high ratios, ranging from 169:100,000 to 197:100,000, was found in the region extending from Ohio and Kentucky through Arkansas and Oklahoma. A ratio of 255:100,000 was found in California, and there were 270 physicians per 100,000 population in Colorado.

Thus, even during a period characterized by a surplus of physicians, it is evident that their distribution varied widely from state to state. Still, there was no agreement about the correct number of physicians for a given population. The Flexner Report had recommended 1 physician for each 1,000 rural residents (a ratio of 100:100,000) and 1 for each 2,000 urban residents (50:100,000). In 1933 the Committee on Costs of Medical Care acknowledged the existing wide range of physicians-to-population ratios and recognized that the real need for service would not necessarily be the same in all states. This committee reported that the need would vary according to the physical condition of the people, as influenced by climate and occupational variations, age and racial composition of the population, and the extent to which preventive medicine was already effectively employed. Despite these admitted problems, the committee arrived at a ratio of 83:100,000 in the (undefined) "standard" community as adequate for diagnosis and treatment of disease. Using data from 1927, the committee concluded that only five states (Montana, North Carolina, South Carolina, Idaho, and North Dakota) fell below the prescribed ratio. Further, the committee rather curiously concluded, "there is no reason to suppose that any shortage of physicians is apparent, even in the state with the smallest relative number of physicians, for even there the effective demand for their services is certainly less than the estimated need."

1936. Though the number of physicians in the United States was about 163,000 in 1936, the physicians-to-population ratio had decreased from 152:100,000 in 1906 to 128:100,000—still well above the ratio (83:100,000) recommended by the Committee on Medical Costs. As in 1906, the South had the majority of states with the lowest ratios (Figure 12.2). South Carolina had only 72 physicians per 100,000 people, and Alabama had only 73, closely followed by North Carolina (with a ratio of 74:100,000) and Mississippi (75:100,000). By 1936, however, Louisiana, Georgia, and especially Florida had increased their physicians-to-population ratios sufficiently to remove them from the lowest category. Other states in this lowest category included Maine (with a ratio of only 58:100,000), North Dakota (75:100,000), South Dakota (81:100,000), and Idaho (84:100,000).

Many states contiguous to the Deep South also had very low physicians-to-population ratios. These included Louisiana (101:100,000), Arkansas (93:100,000), Tennessee (103:100,000), Kentucky (96:100,000), Virginia (102:100,000), and West Virginia (98:100,000). At the other end of the physicians-to-population ratio spectrum, the states with the highest ratios included New York (186:100,000), Colorado (181:100,000), and California (179:100,000). The upper midwestern states of Minnesota, Wisconsin, Iowa, Michigan, and Indiana had moderate physicians-to-population ratios ranging from 110:100,000 to 127:100,000. The most consistent pattern of physician distribution from 1906 through 1936 appears to be the low ratios of the southeastern states. Higher-income states (e.g., California and New York) had higher-than-average rates.

In 1948 a very different perspective on physician supply and levels of adequacy was reported to the President in *The Nation's Health*. In this report, the National Health Assembly suggested that a realistic standard for physicians-to-population ratios should be based on the levels of physicians attained by the top quartile of states. In this group, the average physicians-to-population ratio was 150:100,000—almost double the recommendation of only 15 years earlier! Using this figure, it was estimated that the nation had only about 80 percent of the physicians it needed and, further, that the current distribution of physicians reflected the distribution of social and economic advantage.

The National Health Assembly reported that by 1960 the nation would need 254,000 physicians but would have a supply of only 212,000, and made an urgent plea that U.S. medical schools increase their production of physicians.

1967. By 1967 the number of physicians in the United States was almost 267,000, and yet the physicians-to-population ratio average had increased to only 135:100,000. The familiar pattern of low physicians-to-population ratios continued in the South in 1967 (Figure 12.3). However, the upper midwestern and mountain states also had low ratios. In 1967, Mississippi had the lowest ratio, only 78:100,000. It was closely followed by Alabama (82:100,000) and South Carolina (86:100,000). South Dakota, with a ratio of only 83:100,000, was in the lowest tier of states. Fewer than 100 physicians per 100,000 population were found in Idaho, Nevada, Iowa, New Mexico, Indiana, Kentucky, and West Virginia as well. New York (with a ratio of 207:100,000), Connecticut (177:100,000), and California (170:100,000) had the highest ratios in 1967. The largest cluster of lowest ratios was located in the upper midwestern and mountain states. This represented a shift from the earlier pattern dominated by deficiencies

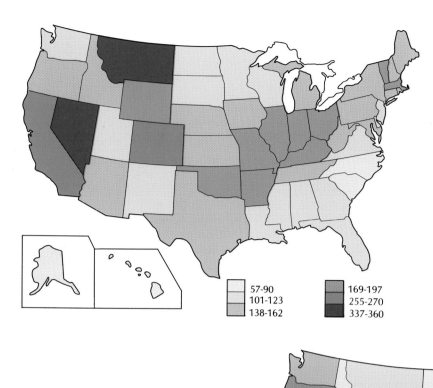

FIGURE 12.1
Physicians per 100,000 Persons, 1906

57-90	169-197
101-123	255-270
138-162	337-360

FIGURE 12.2
Physicians per 100,000 Persons, 1936

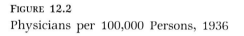

58-84	131-149
90-105	163-186
110-127	318

in the southeastern states, both because of population losses due to migration out of these states and because of migration of physicians to coastal areas.

In 1960 it was estimated that by 1975 the nation would need 330,000 physicians, with an annual medical school graduation rate of 11,000. Thus there was continued pressure to produce more physicians by increasing the capacity of medical schools. Indeed, in 1965 it was suggested that it was probably not possible in the U.S. to educate as many physicians as really needed. In 1970 the Carnegie Commission on Higher Education expressed urgency regarding the serious physician shortage. Despite increased levels of production, the numbers of physicians still fell short of what it was thought the nation needed.

In 1980, however, a 4-year study, the Reports of the Graduate Medical Education National Advisory Committee (GMENAC), the most comprehensive and extensive reports ever completed on physician demography, projected the nation's need for physicians through 1990. The major conclusion was that the nation would be faced with a surplus of practicing physicians, rather than a shortage, and that the surplus would be between 45,700 and 94,350 physicians. Somehow, the physician shortage had turned into a surplus almost overnight! Estimates for the year 2000 were even worse. The required number of physicians was placed at 493,000 and the most reasonable estimate of the number of physicians at 643,000—an excess of 150,000. Thus the nation moved from a physicians-to-

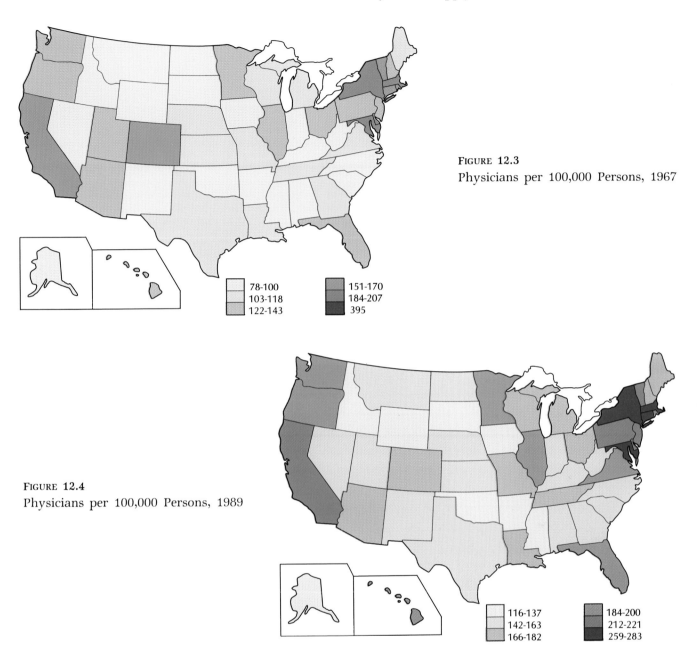

FIGURE 12.3
Physicians per 100,000 Persons, 1967

78-100	151-170
103-118	184-207
122-143	395

FIGURE 12.4
Physicians per 100,000 Persons, 1989

116-137	184-200
142-163	212-221
166-182	259-283

population ratio of 140:100,000 in 1950 to 200:100,000 in 1980 to between 240:100,000 and 280:100,000 by the end of the twentieth century. Needless to say, the argument about whether the United States is faced with a glut or shortage of physicians continues. However, relatively accurate information on the 1989 distribution is available.

1989. Based on the preliminary estimates of state populations in the 1990 Census and on data from the American Medical Association, the distribution of current physicians-to-population ratios is presented in Figure 12.4. In 1989 the total number of practicing physicians was approximately 469,000, and the physicians-to-population ratio was 190:100,000. This

ratio was certainly lower than that projected by the GMENAC study.

Of states with the lowest physicians-to-population ratios, only one, Mississippi (119:100,000) was located in the Southeast. The bulk of states with the lowest physicians-to-population ratios (116:100,000 to 137:100,000) were found distributed across the northern Midwest and the mountain states; they included Iowa (137:100,000), South Dakota (132:100,000), Wyoming (126:100,000), and Idaho (116:100,000). Idaho had the lowest ratio of any state, and Alaska (118:100,000), had the second lowest.

The states with the highest physicians-to-population ratios were concentrated in the Northeast. They included New York (275:100,000), Maryland

(274:100,000) Connecticut (259:100,000), and Massachusetts (283:100,000), which had the highest ratio. Other states in the Northeast, including Vermont, Pennsylvania, and New Jersey, also had very high physicians-to-population ratios, ranging from 212:100,000 to 221:100,000. In the far West, California had the highest ratio (217:100,000).

Generally, with exceptions such as Minnesota, it appeared that states west of the Mississippi and east of the Rocky Mountains comprised the largest group of states with the lowest physicians-to-population ratios.

Conclusion

Too many? Too few? Just enough? Throughout the twentieth century the question of what constitutes the correct number of physicians has apparently puzzled physician groups, health services researchers and planners, the public, and the body politic. Through the years, the pendulum of majority opinion swung from oversupply to undersupply; apparently it has now returned to oversupply. It will continue to swing during the remainder of this century and into the next.

Within several decades, from the mid to the late twentieth century, there has been a revolution in the provision of medical care, from both the scientific and the supply perspectives. Yet the problem of maldistribution of physicians continues. In this chapter we have presented characteristics of the distribution of physicians from state to state. Certain sections of the country have been traditionally undersupplied with physicians, as measured against the national average. At the same time, some states appear to be oversupplied, using the same standard. Again, it is difficult to draw direct conclusions about the variable distribution of physicians and the health of any population because of the complex nature of the relationship alluded to at the beginning of this chapter. In addition to variations in physicians-to-population ratios from state to state, there are major inner city–outer city differences in these ratios. During the first half of the twentieth century, great concern was directed toward the depletion of physicians, especially primary physicians, in the rural areas of many states. Since about 1950, however, an additional concern has been the depletion of physician resources in the low-income and minority sections of many of the larger U.S. cities. In each instance, inevitably the concern is directed toward the relative accessibility of physician services. It is apparent that this problem will continue and perhaps become even more critical during the remainder of the twentieth century.

13

Dentist Supply and Distribution

Dentistry is the healing art concerned with the health of the mouth, especially the teeth. Throughout most of the history of dentistry, the three major conditions which received the most attention were dental caries (or decay of the teeth) and its consequences; disease of the supporting structures of the teeth, including the bones and the gums; and malpositioning of teeth. It is important to note that prior to 1910 preventive dentistry was not emphasized. Doing fillings and extractions, which are almost painless today but were very painful in earlier periods, was the major occupation of dentists during the major portion of this century.

For dentists, as for physicians, there has never been either an accurate assessment or a general consensus concerning an appropriate number of practitioners needed in relation to the population. A factor that may compound the problem of determining such statistics is the unevenness of access to both dentists and physicians caused by financial inequities. Compared to the percentage of the population who are covered to some extent by private or public medical care insurance, a relatively small percentage of people in the United States have insurance to cover the costs of dental care.

Another major factor in determining the variable supply of dentists may be traced to efforts to control dental caries by means of chemical substances, principally fluorides, beginning in 1936. Sodium fluoride is now added to the drinking water supplies of most communities. Though debate continues pertaining to its long-term health effects, this measure is estimated to have reduced the incidence of caries by at least 60 percent. Fluorides have also been added to most dental cleansers, and periodic public programs of topical application take place in many community school systems. Thus, caries and related extractions, the major components of dental practice throughout the first half of the twentieth century, have been drastically reduced, leading to a sharply reduced demand for dental services and dentists.

Geographic Patterns of Dentist Distribution

The first dental school in the United States was opened in 1839. By 1850, there were an estimated 3,000 dentists in the country. By 1900, there were almost 30,000 dentists, or about 1 dentist for every 2,700 people. By 1928, the number of dentists had more than doubled to over 64,000, and there was 1 dentist for every 1,870 people in the United States. About 25 years later, in 1952, though the number of dentists had increased to over 86,000, there was still only 1 dentist for every 1,810 people. With over 128,000 practicing dentists in 1991, there was 1 dentist for approximately every

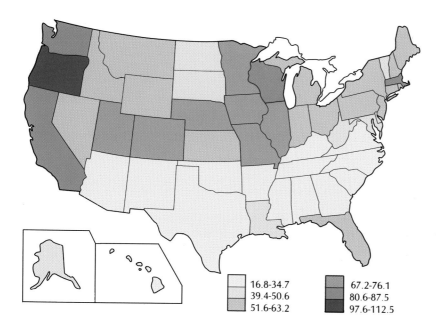

FIGURE **13.1**

Dentists per 100,000 Persons, 1928

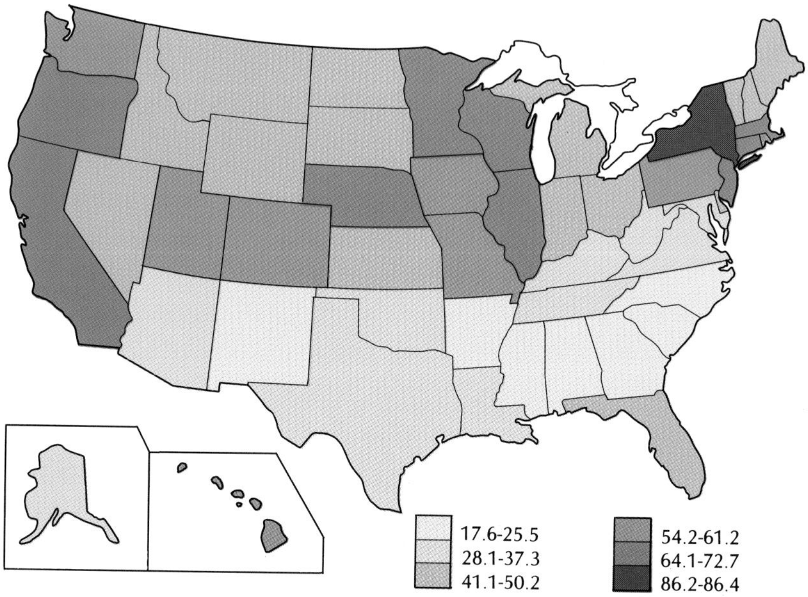

16.8-34.7	67.2-76.1
39.4-50.6	80.6-87.5
51.6-63.2	97.6-112.5

FIGURE **13.2**

Dentists per 100,000 Persons, 1952

17.6-25.5	54.2-61.2
28.1-37.3	64.1-72.7
41.1-50.2	86.2-86.4

1,950 people. In terms of dentists per 100,000 population, the ratio was about 40:100,000 in 1900, and it increased to 55:100,000 in 1928. The ratio stabilized and then even declined, to about 51:100,000 in 1969. In 1987, the most recent date for which information on the number of dentists by state is available, the ratio had declined even further, to about 46:100,000.

1928. As with other indices of access to medical care, such as physicians and hospital beds, a core of southern states, in this instance led by Mississippi, has had the lowest dentists-to-population ratios. In 1928, Mississippi had only 17 dentists per 100,000 population, or 1 dentist for every 6,000 people (Figure 13.1). In this respect, Mississippi appeared to be in a class by itself,

though other states in the region were also distinguished by low ratios. For example, neighboring Alabama had a ratio of 23:100,000, or about 1 dentist for every 4,400 people. Mississippi's neighbor to the west, Arkansas, had a ratio of 24:100,000. South Carolina had 26:100,000, and North Carolina had 28:100,000. The only comparable state outside this region was New Mexico, which had a ratio of 24:100,000. Dentists-to-population ratios were slightly better in surrounding states, such as Georgia (30:100,000) and Tennessee (33:100,000). Farther south, Louisiana had a ratio of 41:100,000 and Florida had 52:100,000.

States with the highest or most favorable dentists-to-population ratios in 1928 were found on both coasts as well as in the Midwest. Oregon had a ratio of almost

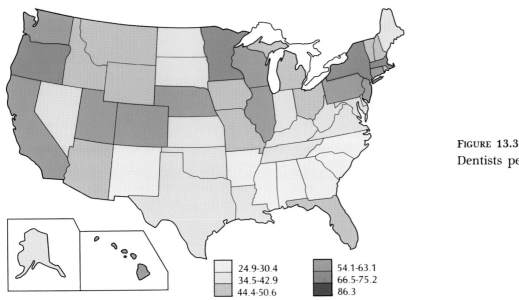

FIGURE **13.3**
Dentists per 100,000 Persons, 1969

24.9-30.4	54.1-63.1
34.5-42.9	66.5-75.2
44.4-50.6	86.3

FIGURE **13.4**
Dentists per 100,000 Persons, 1987

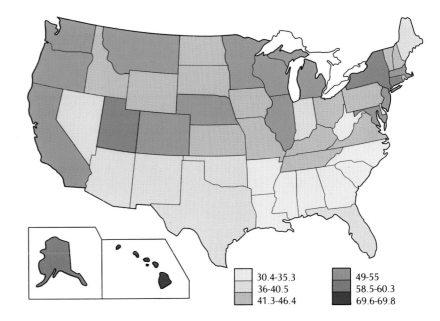

30.4-35.3	49-55
36-40.5	58.5-60.3
41.3-46.4	69.6-69.8

100:100,000, the highest ratio in 1928. Also on the West Coast, California had 88:100,000 and Washington had 84:100,000. In the Midwest, Wisconsin had the most favorable ratio, 81:100,000, while Minnesota had 76:100,000, Colorado 74:100,000, and Nebraska 73:100,000. In the East, Massachusetts had 82:100,000.

Figures for 1952 indicate that in many states population growth had outpaced growth in the supply of dentists. Though several states had experienced considerable increases in dentists-to-population ratios, stable and even decreasing ratios were common.

1952. Unfortunately, most of the states which had the lowest ratios in 1928 had the same or even lower ratios in 1952 (Figure 13.2). Mississippi did improve to

22:100,000. South Carolina had the lowest ratio, having decreased from 26:100,000 in 1928 to 18:100,000 in 1952. In Georgia during the same time period, the ratio fell from 30:100,000 to 24:100,000, and in North Carolina, it fell from 28:100,000 to 24:100,000. In Alabama and Arkansas, the ratios remained stable from 1928 to 1952, at about 24:100,000.

A considerable downward shift in ratios was apparent on the West Coast, where California decreased from 88:100,000 to 64:100,000, Oregon from 98:100,000 to 68:100,000, and Washington from 84:100,000 to 60:100,000. Similarly, Wisconsin decreased from 81:100,000 to 70:100,000 and Massachusetts from 82:100,000 to 68:100,000. Significant increases occurred in several eastern states. For example, New York had the highest ratio in 1952, having moved from a modest 63:100,000 in 1928 to 86:100,000 in 1952. Neighboring Connecticut moved from a ratio of 54:100,000 to 70:100,000. In the Midwest, Michigan, Ohio, Indiana, Illinois, and Iowa had modestly lower dentists-to-population ratios in 1952 than in 1928. In Alabama and Arkansas, the ratios were virtually the same in 1952 as in 1928, which was also true in North Dakota (44:100,000), Oklahoma (34:100,000), Pennsylvania (58:100,000), Rhode Island (59:100,000), and Texas (30:100,000).

1969. In many states, dentists-to-population ratios continued to decline between 1952 and 1969. A familiar pattern of low dentists-to-population ratios for 1969 is illustrated in Figure 13.3. South Carolina, Mississippi, Alabama, Arkansas, Georgia, North Carolina, and Virginia in the South and New Mexico in the West dominated the pattern, with ratios of between 25:100,000 and 30:100,000. As in 1952, New York again had the most favorable ratio, though its ratio had declined to 75:100,000. Also in the East, Massachusetts had a high ratio of 67:100,000. In the Midwest, Minnesota and Wisconsin with 69:100,000 and Nebraska with 61:100,000 had the most favorable ratios. In the far West, high ratios were found in Oregon (73:100,000) and Washington (63:100,000).

1987. By 1987, a substantial reduction had occurred in the range of dentists-to-population ratios from state to state (Figure 13.4). Whereas in 1929 the ratios had ranged from 17:100,000 in Mississippi to 98:100,000 in Oregon, by 1952 the range had decreased somewhat from 18:100,000 in South Carolina to 86:100,000 in New York. In 1969, the ratios had ranged from 25:100,000 in South Carolina to 75:100,000 in New York. However, by 1987 the lowest ratio was again found in Mississippi, which had 30:100,000. The highest ratio in 1987 was that of Hawaii, 70:100,000. In the continental United States, the maximum ratio of 60:100,000 was found in Utah, Connecticut, and New York.

The lowest ratios of between 30:100,000 and 35:100,000 people were found in Mississippi, South Carolina, North Carolina, Alabama, and Arkansas. However, Delaware (with 35:100,000), Indiana (36:100,000), Texas (37:100,000), and Oklahoma (38:100,000) also had dentists-to-population ratios of under 40:100,000. With the exception of Hawaii (70:100,000), the highest dentists-to-population ratios ranged between 55:100,000 and 60:100,000. The states with these high ratios included Utah and Connecticut (60:100,000); Alaska and New York (59:100,000); and Colorado, New Jersey, and Oregon (each with 55:100,000). In the period 1969–1987, 27 of the 50 states had experienced decreases in dentists-to-population ratios, 15 had had increases, and 8 had remained virtually the same.

Conclusion

The twentieth century has seen significant changes in the supply of dentists and in their distribution in the United States. The first several decades of the century were characterized by a supply of dentists that was increasing faster than the population, with resultant increases in dentists-to-population ratios. During the past 50 years, however, the number of dentists per 100,000 population has been stabilizing and even decreasing. As mentioned earlier, this trend may be due to a decreased demand for dental services related primarily to a decrease in dental caries as a result of fluoridation in public water supplies. The decreasing number of people who are expected to need dental repairs in the future may indicate that there will be further decreases in the demand for dentists. However, there is a considerable unmet demand in the population, especially among the uninsured poor, who generally receive only emergency dental care. Should circumstances change and greater access to dental care be accorded to this population, the country could experience at least a short-term increase in the demand for dental services and care.

Distribution of Hospitals

14

To most people, the hospital and the medical care resources associated with it represent the pinnacle of available medical care. Physically as well as symbolically, today's hospitals contain personnel and facilities at the forefront of modern scientific medicine. Most people turn to hospitals in the belief that they offer the best chance of recovery from serious illness or accident. As recently as 1955, however, the statement was made, "Within living memory an age-old institution has been transformed from a hostel for the sick-poor into a medical center for everyone." During most of the nineteenth century, the large majority of hospitals were charitable institutions which treated only poor unfortunates who were unable to afford treatment in their homes. As late as 1877 in the United States, it was suggested that hospital care be limited to individuals who had no homes and to the poor who could afford home health care.

Indeed, it is instructive to note that, until 1836, patients admitted to St. Bartholomew Hospital in London were required to deposit or give security in the amount of 17s. 6d. to cover burial expenses in the event of death. Such a practice certainly did not inspire confidence among the general populace and particularly not among potential patients. Today in the United States opinions about hospitals continue to evolve. Some critics decry the "medicalization of society" and criticize the hospital as the purveyor and controller of medical care.

The Early Hospital Experience

The first general hospital in the American colonies was Pennsylvania Hospital of Philadelphia, chartered in 1751. This was followed by New York Hospital, which was chartered in 1773 but, due to the Revolution, not opened until 1791. Massachusetts General Hospital in Boston admitted its first patients in 1821. Each of these hospitals was located on a "healthyful," open, airy, and elevated site, away from the center of the nearby city. These locations were chosen in part to ensure the health of patients through the "enjoyment of fresh and salubrious breezes" but also because hospitals were considered noxious and disagreeable places which no one would want to live near.

Hospital Growth in the United States

While asylums for the mentally ill proliferated during the early and middle parts of the nineteenth century, the building of general hospitals in the United States during the period appears to have been quite limited. A clear assessment of the situation is difficult to achieve because of the lack of aggregate data on hospitals of the period. The first "complete" census of hospitals was accomplished in 1909. At that time the nation had 4,359 hospitals with a total bed capacity of 421,000. By 1920, however, the number of general and specialty hospitals had declined to 4,013 and the number of beds to just over 311,000. This averages out to about 2.9 hospital beds for every 1,000 persons in the United States. Twenty years later, in 1940, there were 4,165 nonfederal general hospitals with a total of some 401,209 beds, an average of about 4.7 beds per 1,000 population. It is obvious that the increase in hospital beds outpaced population growth during this period. This pattern shifted somewhat over the next 20 years, and in 1960 there were about 3.7 general hospital beds per 1,000 people. Presently there are about 5,500 nonfederal general short-stay hospitals with approximately 933,000 beds, an average of 3.7 beds per 1,000 persons in the United States. Thus the average number of hospital beds per 1,000 persons in the United States appears to have stabilized. It has been suggested that the hospital beds-to-population ratio may decrease with the closing of many rural community hospitals. The actual current availability of beds is believed to be considerably greater than in the past because of the decreasing average length of stay of patients which has occurred over the past 20 years.

Geographic Patterns in Hospital Bed Distribution

While the national average hospital beds-to-population ratio of approximately 3.7:1,000 is a bit lower than the recommended level of 4.0:1,000 people, it is important to remember, as an analogus, that it would be possible for a person to drown in a stream which had an average depth of 3 feet. That is, while the national average provides a gross measure of availability, the state patterns are more useful as indicators of geographic availability. Historically there has been, and there continues to be today, considerable geographic variation in the distribution of hospital beds across the United States.

1920. In 1920 the number of hospital beds per 1,000 population at the state level ranged from a low of 0.9 in Mississippi to a high of 7.2 in Nevada. The national distribution of hospital beds per 1,000 population in 1920 reflected a pattern of considerable deficit, which was especially noticeable in the southeastern states and extending westward (Figure 14.1). In addition to Mississippi, other southern states were substantially "underbedded" with respect to the availability of general hospitals. Georgia, Florida, Arkansas, North Carolina, South Carolina, Tennessee, and Kentucky all had fewer than 2.0 beds per 1,000 population in 1920. Texas and Oklahoma also fell into this lowest category.

This unfortunate deficit in hospital beds in southern states may reflect the presence of large numbers of blacks, for whom provision of hospital services in 1920 was separate and very unequal in terms of both quality and quantity of care. Generally, there were few hospitals devoted to the care of the black population and few general hospitals that were integrated. In most southern states, the extant hospitals were reserved for exclusive use by the white population.

All the states outside the southeastern and near southwestern states of Arkansas, Texas, and Oklahoma had hospital beds-to-population ratios higher than did the low-ratio states discussed above, though some provided fewer than 2.5 beds per 1,000 population. These states were widely distributed and included Delaware, Idaho, Indiana, Iowa, Kansas, Louisiana, Michigan, Utah, Vermont, Virginia, and West Virginia.

Other states with low ratios of hospital beds per 1,000 population, that is from 2.5 to 2.7:1,000, were found across the United States from coast to coast in 1920. Maine and New Hampshire fell into this category in the Northeast, as did a contiguous cluster of states stretching from Virginia northwestward to Michigan; the four plains states of Iowa, Missouri, Nebraska, and Kansas; and Idaho and Utah in the mountain area. In 1920, a total of 26 states had ratios below the national average of 2.9:1,000.

With the exception of New York state, which had the highest ratio (5.4:1,000), the states with the highest hospital beds-to-population ratios were in the West. These included Wyoming (4.8:1,000), Colorado (5.1:1,000), Arizona (5.2:1,000), and California (4.8:1,000).

As with the distribution of physicians discussed in Chapter 12, the most prominent feature of the distribution of hospital beds in the early part of the century appears to have been the substandard position of most southeastern states as well as of the states extending westward through Texas. Similarly, the western states were among those with the highest ratios.

1930. In 1930, the adequacy of hospital beds for two groups was addressed, specifically farmers and Blacks. Of particular concern for farmers was the distance to the nearest hospital. It was estimated that over one-third of the rural population had to travel at least 20 miles to the nearest hospital, and 38 percent spent at least 1 hour in such travel under the most favorable conditions (that is, in summer). Thus, the condition of rural roads was especially important. In winter the average travel time 'to the nearest hospital was an hour and a half; 15 percent of rural residents reported travel times of 3 or more hours.

The number of hospital beds available to Black people was determined to be far less than their actual needs. In 1930 it was estimated that there were about 7 beds per 1,000 people in the United States, but in the approximately 200 small hospitals that provided care for blacks, there was fewer than 1 bed per 1,000 persons. Truly, the black American was at a particularly severe disadvantage. Though this problem existed in every section of the country, the situation was most extreme in the rural southeastern states, as demonstrated by their low hospital beds-to-population ratios.

While the number of hospitals actually decreased between 1920 and 1930, there was an increase in the number of hospital beds. By 1940, there were 4.7 general hospital beds per 1,000 persons, reflecting a continued increase in the number of hospital beds relative to a very slight increase in the general population during the decade dominated by the Great Depression. Despite these changes, the pattern of hospital beds-to-population ratios of 1940 very closely resembles that of 1920.

1940. Again in 1940, the pattern of states with the lowest hospital beds-to-population ratios was dominated by states in the Southeast as well as Arkansas, Oklahoma, and Texas. The only notable changes included the increase in hospital beds-to-population ratio of Florida and the addition of Indiana to the lowest category (Figure 14.2). The states with the lowest ratios included Mississippi (1.5:1,000), Arkansas (1.8:1,000), and Kentucky (1.9:1,000). Florida, which had only 1.7 beds per 1,000 population in 1920, increased its ratio to 3.3:1,000 in 1940.

Nevada, probably in part because of its low population, stood out in 1940 as the state with the highest hospital beds-to-population ratio, 6.2:1,000. With the exception of Massachusetts (5.2:1,000), the states with the highest hospital beds-to-population ratios were located in the western part of the United States. Montana, with 5.6:1,000, had the highest ratio, and it was closely followed by Wyoming (5.2:1,000), Colorado (5.1:1,000), and California (5.3:1,000). Again, with the exception of California, these high hospital beds-to-population ratios were probably caused by the relatively low total populations of these states; the addition of only a moderate number of hospital beds may have significantly raised the hospital bed-to-population ratios.

Public Law 725, the Federal Hospital Construction Act of 1946, is probably the most important piece of U.S. legislation pertaining to hospitals. Funding provided by this legislation provides financing and support of needs surveys for hospital construction in underserved areas, especially in rural areas and in southern states. In 1949 this act was amended, further increasing the Federal appropriation and share for hospital construction projects. Despite these programs, by 1960 the national average ratio of hospital beds to population had fallen to 3.7:1,000. Obviously, hospital construction and expansion between 1940 and 1960 had not kept pace with the rapid post-World War II population increases. Nevertheless there were some dramatic changes in the ratios of some states, as well as a general increase across the country.

1960. By 1960, only Alaska had fewer than 2.7 beds per 1,000 population (Figure 14.3). As in previous years, the lower hospital beds-to-population ratios were concentrated in the southeastern states, despite some significant individual gains between 1940 and 1960. The following southeastern states had fewer than 3.0 beds per 1,000 persons: Alabama (a ratio of 2.8:1,000), Georgia (2.7:1,000), Mississippi (2.9:1,000, up from 1.5:1,000 in 1940). In addition, Utah (2.8:1,000) and New Mexico (2.8:1,000) had among the lowest ratios in the nation. California, with 3.0 beds per 1,000 persons, was apparently underbedded, or at least it fell into the very low category. In all likelihood, this change in California's ratio was caused by the state's tremendous population increase between 1940 and 1960.

Generally, hospital beds per 1,000 population decreased in most states between 1940 and 1960. In California, for example, the decrease was from a ratio of 5.3:1,000 in 1940 to 3.0:1,000 in 1960. Arizona decreased from 4.9:1,000 to 3.2:1,000 during the same period, and Nevada declined from 6.2:1,000 to 4.2:1,000. Again, these rather large decreases were probably caused by the increases in population in southwestern states between 1940 and 1960.

A small cluster of states, including Montana, Wyoming, South Dakota, and Delaware, had the highest ratios, from 4.8:1,000 to 5.3:1,000. States in the very high ratio category, that is, from 4.3:1,000 to 4.5:1,000, included Vermont and New Hampshire in the Northeast, as well as West Virginia, Wisconsin, and North Dakota.

Also apparent was a decrease in the range of hospital beds-to-population ratios between 1920 and 1960. The range in 1920 was 63; by 1940, the range had decreased to 4.2, and in 1960 it was only 3.1. Thus it appeared that, despite continued variations, the states were becoming more uniform in their distribution of hospital beds-to-population ratios. Indeed, 28 states had ratios ranging from 3.2:1,000 to 4.2:1,000 in 1960.

In 1975 the National Health Planning and Resources Development Act explicitly stated, "There should be less than four non-federal, short-term hospital beds per 1,000 persons in a health service area, except under extraordinary circumstances." Moreover, the Secretary of Health indicated that areas with ratios lower than 4:1,000 persons but higher than 3.7:1,000 should

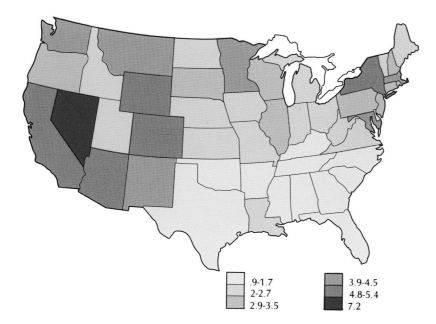

FIGURE **14.1**

General Hospital Beds per 1,000 Persons, 1920

FIGURE **14.2**

General Hospital Beds per 1,000 Persons, 1940

strongly attempt to decrease their ratios toward the lower figure. Thus, with hospital beds as with physicians, an attempt was made to standardize medical resources to a normative level of medical care provision.

At the state level in 1960, therefore, according to the 3.7:1,000 ratio, 22 states were considered "over-bedded."

1989. Obviously, when viewed from the current perspective and at the state level, the 1975 recommendation of 3.7 beds per 1,000 population had little impact, at least in the longer run (Figure 14.4). In 1989, for example, 16 states had ratios of over 4.0:1,000 compared to 17:1,000 in 1960. The highest ratios, from 4.2:1,000 to 5:1,000, were found primarily in a group of states in

the central portion of the United States, extending from the northern boundary abutting Canada to the Gulf of Mexico—a very radical departure from the earlier patterns.

Most noticeably different in 1989 was the concentration of some of the highest hospital beds-to-population ratios in the Southeast. Of particular interest was Mississippi, which had a ratio of 4.6:1,000, compared to 2.9:1,000 in 1960. Alabama, Arkansas, and Tennessee had ratios of at least 4.2:1,000, placing them in the highest category. Other southern states, including Georgia, Kentucky, and Louisiana, were in the very high category, with ratios from 3.8:1,000 to 4.1:1,000. The highest ratios continued northwestward through Missouri, Iowa, Kansas, and the Dakotas. West Vir-

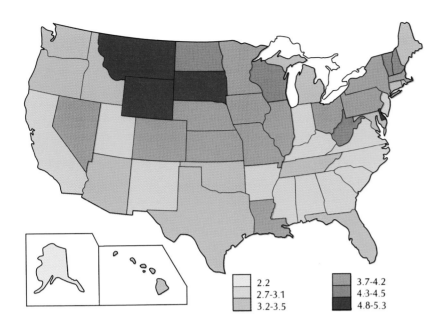

FIGURE **14.3**
General Hospital Beds per 1,000
Persons, 1960

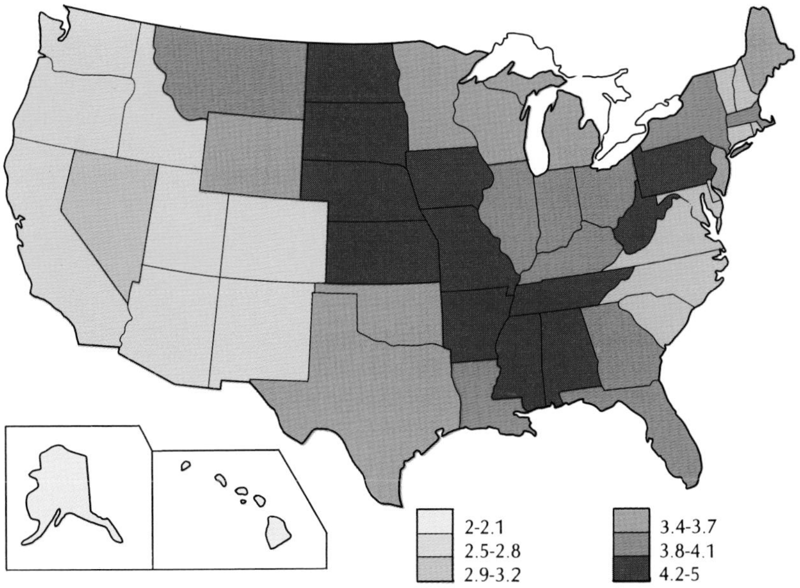

2.2		3.7-4.2
2.7-3.1		4.3-4.5
3.2-3.5		4.8-5.3

FIGURE **14.4**
General Hospital Beds per 1,000
Persons, 1989

2-2.1		3.4-3.7
2.5-2.8		3.8-4.1
2.9-3.2		4.2-5

ginia and Pennsylvania were also in the highest category.

States in the next highest category, that is, with ratios of from 3.4:1,000 to 3.7:1,000, were widely distributed, from Montana in the West; to Texas and Oklahoma in the Southwest; to Michigan, Wisconsin, and Minnesota in the Midwest; and to New Jersey and Maine in the Northeast.

The newest states, Alaska and Hawaii, had the lowest hospital beds-to-population ratios, 2.1:1,000 and 2:1,000, respectively. Other states with low ratios were located in the Southwest and the far West. States with ratios between 2.5:1,000 and 2.8:1,000 included Washington, Oregon, California, Utah, Arizona, Colorado, and New Mexico.

The reasons for this radical change in the geographic pattern of hospital beds per population were complex. In the rural plains—that is, in states such as the Dakotas, Kansas, Iowa, and Missouri—the higher ratios may have been due to a combination of hospital construction and relatively stable or even declining populations in predominantly rural areas. In states such as Pennsylvania and West Virginia, hospital construction had been supported by federal agencies and by national organizations, such as the United Mine Workers, to service their member populations. The lower ratios in the far West and in the Southwest again may have been due in part to recent trends in migration and to proportionately large population increases. Whatever the reasons, a regional consolidation of hospital beds-to-population ratios appears to have taken place between 1960 and 1989.

Conclusion

Patterns of hospital provision, while appearing to be relatively stable in the short run, have actually significantly been altered through the addition and deletion of facilities, shifts in population, and government intervention with funding and building programs. This has obviously been true for the United States during the twentieth century. As attitudes toward hospital care changed, and as insurance plans for subsidizing hospital care costs developed among the middle and lower socioeconomic classes, demands for hospital facilities increased. Though broad southeastern sections of the country began the twentieth century with well below average levels of hospital bed provision, in part due to a legacy of racial discrimination, it appears that most states had adequate levels of hospital beds by 1989. On the other hand, perhaps related to more recent trends in migration, states in the far West and the Southwest had very low hospital beds-to-population ratios. Overall, however, the gap in hospital beds per 1,000 population between the highest-ratio and the lowest-ratio states decreased significantly, from 6.3 in 1920 to only 3.0 in 1989. Thus it appeared that, with the reduction in the difference between the highest and lowest hospital beds-to-population ratios, the states were moving toward a common ratio, despite the complexity of underlying factors related to the provision of hospital beds across the nation. It will be interesting to see whether this trend continues in the near future.

15

Distribution of Mental Health Care

In the United States during the twentieth century, probably no other sector of medical care has changed as radically as mental health care. Some of the most fundamental changes have occurred over the past 40 years in terms of the locations in which mental health care is provided. For a number of reasons, many public "insane asylums," or long-term mental health hospitals, have been evacuated and closed. These traditional institutional settings for mental health care were replaced by a movement in the 1960s to provide care in the community. It is generally acknowledged that in the United States, historically and presently, mental health care has been and continues to be woefully inadequate and ineffective, no matter where it is provided. The origins of the institutional and community mental health care approaches are presented below, in conjunction with descriptions of the resulting changes in the distribution of care.

Historical Origins

The Eighteenth Century

The mental health care situation in the United States in 1900 had its origins in changes which took place in the nineteenth century and even earlier. In the Colonial and immediate post-Colonial periods, mental illness was not at all understood. Little if any hope was held out for victims. Their afflictions were believed to be caused by "acts of God" or, conversely, by demoniacal possession or witchcraft. Nevertheless, several "scientific" treatments were devised, prescribed, and applied by a small group of physicians and others who believed the sources of mental illness to be physical. For example, bloodletting was very popular. "Black bile" was purportedly responsible for manic-depressive syndromes; by bleeding the patient, the offending humor could be literally drained from the body, resulting in cure for the patient. Bloodletting was accomplished by actually lancing veins; by applying leeches to particular parts of the body (around the anus was prescribed for melancholia); and by "cupping," a process in which a hot glass cup was applied to the shaved head (or other presumably afflicted area) to draw blood away from internal parts of the body. Some such practitioners thought that "new blood would make a new man," and consequently transfusions were used. Unfortunately, the blood frequently used was that of calves or lambs; this often led to the death of the patient, who, according to current standards, might more aptly be called "the victim."

Shock treatments were used to expel evil spirits and jolt the patient back to reality. Flogging, purging, and induced vomiting were the most common shock treatments administered. Whippings and cold showers lasting up to 20 minutes were also advocated. In a "bath of surprise," the patient was induced to stand or sit, unknowingly, upon a trapdoor that concealed a large tub of very cold water. At the appropriate time, as determined by the therapist, the trapdoor was opened and the patient plunged into the tub. Other such surprises consisted of boats constructed to break apart, forcing patients to swim to shore in cold water, and bridges designed to collapse as patients walked across them.

Benjamin Rush, a physician who signed the Declaration of Independence, contrived a "gyrator." This machine consisted of a board to which the patient was strapped, feet to the center, and whirled, much as if on a children's merry-go-round, at high rates of speed, causing the blood to rush to the head. This treatment was viewed as a form of stimulus and was administered to patients stricken with "lethargy."

The Nineteenth Century

Given the state of the art of treatment for mental illness during the eighteenth century, it is perhaps fortunate that there were few hospitals for the mentally ill. The first hospital designed solely for the mentally ill was a facility in Williamsburg, Virginia, which was opened in 1773. This remained the only state hospital of its kind in the country until the Eastern Lunatic Asylum was opened in 1824 at Lexington, Kentucky. This situation changed relatively rapidly, however, and the period 1820–1870 may be characterized as the "golden age" of public insane asylums in the United States. By 1860, 28 of the (then) 33 states had at least one public mental hospital. The impetus for this building movement was derived from several sources, including: the emerging belief that insanity was substantially on the increase and was a threat to society; the belief and mounting "evidence" that insanity was inherently curable; and the effectiveness of Dorothea Dix (1802–1887), a champion of humane medical care for the insane.

Concomitant with the mounting perception of an increase in the incidence and prevalence of insanity was diffusion and acceptance of the belief that insanity could be readily cured if treated properly. Americans in the Jacksonian era, no longer content with divine explanations of mental illness, began intensive inquiries into the origins of the disease. By 1852, for example, some 184 causes of mental illness had been identified and classified. These causes included physical diseases such as yellow fever, scarlet fever, and measles. "Such quaint views as suppression of perspiration" and "suppression of hemorrhoids" were also thought to lead to disturbance of the brain. Other supposed physical causes included "bathing in cold water" and "sleeping in a barn with new hay." Among moral causes of insanity were "preaching sixteen days and nights" and "study excessive" (with which many students might concur). In retrospect, many of these alleged specific causes of mental illness seem silly and unscientific. Nevertheless, they may have been of value at the time, in that they represented a radical revision of prevailing medical opinion regarding the origins of mental illness.

Equally important, it became accepted both in the medical community and among the general population that mental illness could be cured regardless of the specific cause. What was thought essential to effecting a cure was prompt removal of the patient from the stress and strain of home and community living to the sanctuary of the asylum, with its simple and rigid routine. Thus, mere removal to the asylum, a change in location, was believed to be sufficient in many cases to "secure the beginning of convalescence and not unfrequently [an] improvement in behavior and conversation." (As we shall show below, a reversal of this thinking was partly responsible for the community mental health care movement of the mid-twentieth century.)

Impetus for the development and construction of many insane asylums in both the United States and Western Europe was embodied in a single person, Dorothea Dix. A retired schoolteacher living in Boston, she was appalled at the living conditions of a group of mentally ill persons she observed while teaching Sunday school in a local jail. This experience led her to begin a new career in 1841, which was to last some 40 years. Dix was dedicated to exposing the miserable conditions of the mentally ill who were confined in rooms, sheds, or prison dungeons. She lobbied effectively with state legislatures across the country for the establishment of state-supported asylums. An estimated 20 states responded directly to her appeals, and several states credited more than one institution to her efforts. Dix spent her last years in a home on the grounds of an asylum in Trenton, New Jersey. Upon her death in 1887, the superintendent of Bloomingdale Hospital wrote, "Thus has died and been laid to rest, in the most quiet, unostentatious way, the most useful and distinguished woman America has yet produced." Dorothea Dix was buried in a cemetery near Boston, Massachusetts.

During this golden age of asylums in the United States, the mentally ill were increasingly removed from their homes and local communities and transferred, at times great distances, to relatively large and geographically isolated facilities. This pattern was to persist well into the twentieth century, when extreme changes in geographic strategies related to mental health care took place.

As mentioned previously, belief in the curability of the insane was the cornerstone of the rise and proliferation of state-supported asylums. There developed what amounted to a cult of curability, a general conviction that mental illness was curable, especially if treated early. The percentage of cures in annual reports from asylums began to rise. Cure rates, based upon the number of persons released from an asylum each year, increased rapidly to 80 and 90 percent. In 1842 in Virginia a recovery rate of 100 percent was reported, excluding patients who had died in treatment. In 1843, the annual report of the Ohio State Lunatic Asylum at Columbus stated, as a matter of fact and without exception, "percent of recovery on all recent cases discharged this year, 100."

But all was not well. Careful readers of the reports and the accompanying statistics became skeptics. As early as 1842, for example, a physician observed that the only measure of recovery was release from the asylum. It was therefore possible for an individual to be counted as recovered any number of times. In Pennsylvania, for example, 87 persons contributed to 274 recoveries. In New York one woman was discharged as recovered 6 times in one year. Ultimately, she was reported to have been "cured" no fewer than 46 times before her death—which occurred in a hospital for the insane!

Enthusiasm for cure and percentages of recovery plummeted quickly. By the 1870s, reports of less than 20 percent recovery rates were common. At one asylum in Michigan in 1884, the recovery rate was placed at 9.77 percent. At the McClean Asylum in Massachusetts in 1840, it was observed that "all cases, certainly recent . . . recover under a fair trial." Some 17 years later, the same superintendent wrote, "I have come to the conclusion, that when a man once becomes insane, he is about used up for this world." State asylums and hospitals for the insane were thus transformed from "a class of noble structures which had arisen throughout the land" to being considered at best massive warehouses for the incurable mentally ill. However, no alternative was available for the mentally ill. While new construction of large and remote asylums slowed, the institutions which were already in existence were substantially increased in size to accommodate the demand for storage of the country's mentally ill. It was this legacy that was carried into the twentieth century.

Geographic Patterns in the Distribution of Mental Health Care

1903. In 1903 there were approximately 145,000 patients, or about 180 per 100,000 population, in mental hospitals distributed throughout the United States (Graph: Number and Ratio of Patients in State and County Mental Hospitals). As depicted in Figure 15.1, the ratio varied considerably among the states, ranging from only 48:100,00 in Arkansas to 472:100,000 in Nevada. Ratios of 100:100,000 and lower were found in a significant cluster in the Southeast and extending westward. The lowest ratios extended almost uninterrupted, with the exception of Georgia and Florida, from North Carolina and South Carolina to Alabama, Louisiana, Mississippi, Arkansas, Texas, Oklahoma, and New Mexico. The pattern of relative "underservice" with regard to the provision of long-term mental hospital beds in the southeastern states was similar to the patterns for physicians and dentists discussed in Chapters 12 and 13. More than likely, this pattern again reflected a failure to provide services for blacks, who constituted a large percentage of the states' populations. Wyoming also had a low ratio, which may have been due in part to its rather late (1890) entry into the United States. Two other states with low ratios, Oklahoma (1907) and New Mexico (1912) also entered late. However, the patient-to-population ratio (166:100,000) in the Arizona territory, which entered at the same time as New Mexico, was almost 3 times higher.

At the other end of the spectrum of care, patient-to-population ratios of approximately 200:100,000 were concentrated in the Northeast, in Rhode Island, New Jersey, Connecticut, Massachusetts, and New York; across the Midwest, in states such as Michigan, Wisconsin, and Minnesota; and along the West Coast from Washington and Oregon to California and Nevada. The high ratios in northeastern and to a lesser extent in midwestern states may have been due in part to these states' relatively long histories of asylum development and incarceration.

1933. Some 30 years later, there were more than 350,000 patients in state and county mental hospitals, over 2.5 times as many as in 1903. Also, the average ratio of patients to population had increased from about 180:100,000 in 1903 to 282:100,000 in 1933, over 1.5 times as high. Thus, though the cult of curability had been buried decades previously, the asylums continued to be enlarged and greater numbers of patients warehoused in them.

In 1933, as in 1903, the largest cluster of underserved states appeared in the Southeast (Figure 15.2). Again the lowest ratios extended from North Carolina and South Carolina westward through Texas, New Mexico, and Utah. However, the lowest ratio was found in New Mexico—157:100,000, almost 3 times higher than the 1903 ratio (55:100,000). In 1903 the lowest ratio (49:100,000) had occurred in Arkansas. Though it was still relatively very low in 1933, the Arkansas' ratio (184:100,000) was almost 4 times higher than it had been around the turn of the century! Such large increases were limited primarily to states at the lower end of the care spectrum.

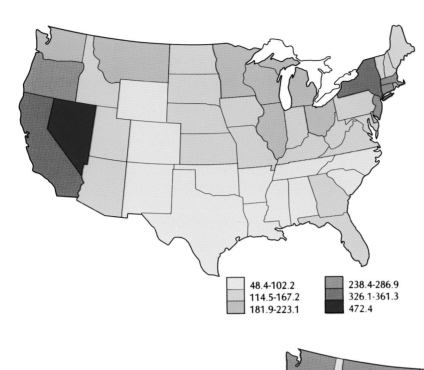

FIGURE 15.1
Patients in Public Mental Hospitals per 100,000 Persons, 1903

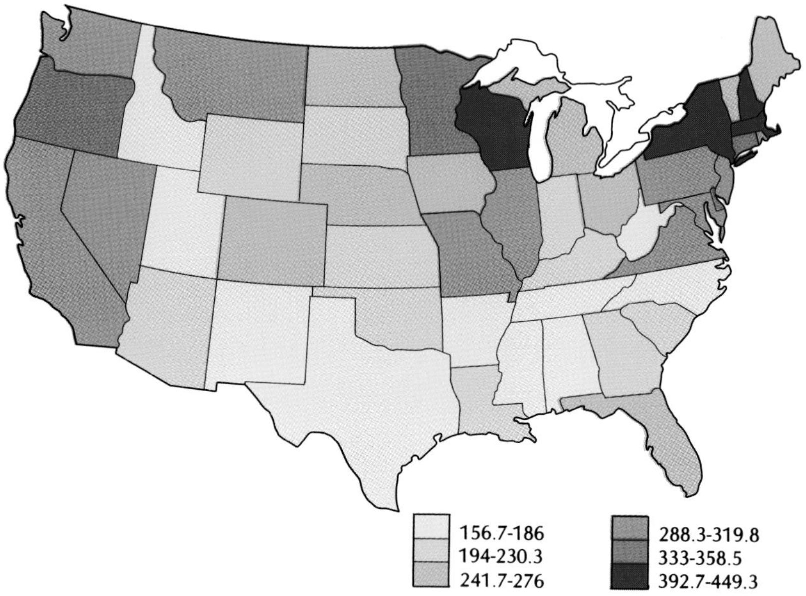

48.4-102.2	238.4-286.9
114.5-167.2	326.1-361.3
181.9-223.1	472.4

FIGURE 15.2
Patients in Public Mental Hospitals per 100,000 Persons, 1933

156.7-186	288.3-319.8
194-230.3	333-358.5
241.7-276	392.7-449.3

Increases in patients-to-population ratios among the states with the highest ratios were not as great. In some instances, such as Nevada and California, the ratios actually declined significantly. In Nevada the 1903 ratio of 472:100,000 was reduced to 314:100,000 in 1933. Similarly, probably reflecting population migration to the Southwest, the ratio in California fell from 361:100,000 in 1903 to 288:100,000 in 1933. The states that showed increases included New York, which increased from 326:100,000 to 431:100,000 population, and Connecticut, which increased from 259:100,000 to 356:100,000.

In 1933 there remained significant clusters of states with high patients-to-population ratios. These in-

cluded Connecticut, New York, and Massachusetts (449:100,000) in the East, and Oregon (339:100,000) and Nevada (314:100,00) in the West.

As mentioned above, the largest increases in patients-to-population ratios occurred among the states in the lower categories. This is reflected in the fact that in 1903 the highest ratio (Nevada, 472:100,00) was 10 times higher than the lowest (Arkansas, 48:100,000). In 1933 the highest ratio (Massachusetts, 449:100,00) was only 3 times higher than the lowest (New Mexico, 157:100,000). Overall, the average patients-to-population ratios in the United States increased from 180:100,000 in 1903 to 283:100,000 in 1933, reflecting the increased predisposition to place the mentally ill in

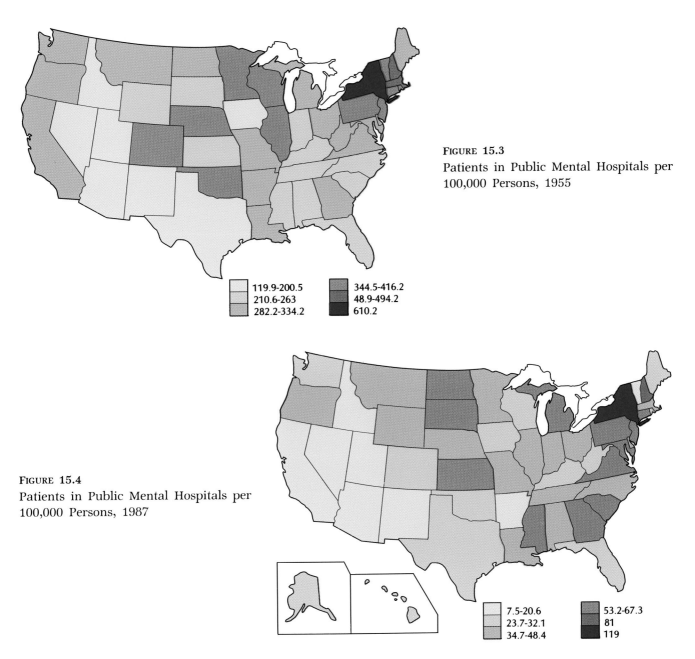

FIGURE 15.3
Patients in Public Mental Hospitals per 100,000 Persons, 1955

119.9-200.5	344.5-416.2
210.6-263	48.9-494.2
282.2-334.2	610.2

FIGURE 15.4
Patients in Public Mental Hospitals per 100,000 Persons, 1987

7.5-20.6	53.2-67.3
23.7-32.1	81
34.7-48.4	119

institutions. Some 22 years later, in 1954, the total number of patients in public state and county hospitals reached its peak.

1955. Between 1903 and 1933, on average, the number of patients in public state and county mental hospitals or asylums increased by 7,000 annually. Between 1933 and 1955, the annual increase averaged over 9,000, and the peak hospital population was about 560,000. In 1933 the national ratio was 282:100,000. By 1955, the ratio had increased to 338:100,000. The peak actually occurred in 1954, when the ratio was 341:100,000.

In terms of the geography of mental health care, it appears the greatest change in distribution was the shift in the cluster of states with the lowest patients-to-population ratios (Figure 15.3). Notably, only Florida, Tennessee, and North Carolina had ratios in the lowest quartile. The bulk of states in this range (from 120:100,000 to 230:100,000) were located in the West and in the Southwest; included were New Mexico, Arizona, Utah, Texas, Idaho, and Wyoming. Interestingly, Nevada was not included among the states with the lowest ratios. It had the highest ratio in 1903 and remained in the highest category in 1933. In fact, 8 of the 12 states in the lowest quartile actually experienced reductions in their patients-to-population ratios between 1933 and 1955. Decreases in these and other states, however, were more than offset by increases in the ratios of some of the leading states. For example, New York moved from a ratio of 431:100,000 in 1933 to 610:100,000 in 1955. During the same period, New Hampshire moved from 383:100,000 to 494:100,000 persons and New Jersey moved from 306:100,000 to 415:100,000. There appears to have been a continued concentration of the highest ratios in the northeastern United States, with Wisconsin, Illinois, and Minnesota making up a secondary cluster in the Midwest.

Changes in Philosophy

The year 1955 represents a watershed in the number of patients in state and county mental hospitals, as it ended a 54-year period of increases. Since then, the total number of patients in these hospitals has declined annually. The figure for 1987 was about 110,000 persons in state and county mental hospitals, a decrease of approximately 450,000, representing an average of more than 20,000 patients per year. Moreover, the peak ratio of 341:100,000 in 1954 had decreased to only 44:100,000 by 1987, a decrease of 77 percent.

By 1955, most patients who had been lobotomized (an extreme form of treatment no longer used) in the 1930s and 1940s were in permanent custodial care. By the late 1970s and 1980s most were dead, causing a numerical drop. Several other factors combined to cause this radical change in the number of patients in public mental hospitals. These reasons include the introduction of psychotropic drugs, the passage of legislation pertaining to the civil rights of patients, public outrage at the conditions of the asylums and hospitals, and a revised philosophy pertaining to the geography of mental health care.

Psychotropic drugs were first introduced into the United States from France in 1954. These drugs were welcomed as relatively simple and effective measures for calming and controlling psychotic patients by suppressing their hallucinations and delusions. Later drug treatments were introduced to control less severe problems and neuroses. Only relatively recently have the negative long-term effects of many of these mind-altering drugs been identified causing considerable rethinking about drug therapy.

It was also in the mid-1950s that civil rights activists began to litigate the right of least restrictive alternative in mental health care. The principle of least restrictive setting was enunciated in an Alabama federal district court case. Lawyers argued that states had an obligation to search for alternatives; to provide care in less restrictive settings; and moreover, to discharge the committed patient outright. This move explicitly focused on removal of patients from large and geographically isolated state mental hospitals to small group residences or other facilities within the community.

These developments coincided with revelations in the mass media of the abysmal conditions in which the mentally ill were kept in asylums and hospitals. Monstrous cases of abuse were documented, and the public became enraged about the treatment of the mentally ill, who had been hidden from public view for well over a century.

Finally, a radical change in philosophy took place within the field of mental health care. It became accepted among mental health professionals that patients could be more effectively treated and would improve more readily within their own communities than in the isolated asylum or hospital setting. It was suggested, in fact, that removal of patients from hospitals would reduce the chronicity of their diseases and improve their chances for cure.

Taken together, these factors provided the foundation for the community mental health movement, the latest philosophy of mental health care. Unfortunately, this movement has been described as only partially successful, at best. Major problems have arisen in many cities because of the long-term effects of psychotropic drugs, the failure of communities to provide adequate residences or halfway houses for patients released from hospitals or in need of professional supervision, public resistance to location of these facilities (the so-called NIMBY—Not In My Back Yard—syndrome) in any but the lowest-income areas of cities, and the failure of the federal government to adequately plan for and provide adequate funding for community mental health centers.

1987. The most recent figures for patients in state and county hospitals reflect the impact of the community mental health movement (Figure 15.4). Many state and county hospitals have been closed and razed. Others have been significantly reduced in size. About 100,000 patients remain in public mental hospitals, a national average of between 40 and 45 patients per 100,000 persons. Unfortunately, former and prospective mental patients are now believed to constitute large segments of the homeless in the United States.

The results of the community mental health movement are obvious in reductions of the observed ratios of patients to population in the various states. In 1955, for example, Arkansas had 287 patients per 100,000 persons in public hospitals. By 1987, the Arkansas ratio had been reduced to only 8:100,000—the lowest ratio in the country. In 1987 the highest ratio was found in New York—119:100,000. This ratio was the same as that of New Mexico in 1955, which at that time was the lowest ratio in the nation. It is also notable that New York was the only state with a ratio higher than 100. The remaining states had ratios of 81:100,000 and below.

Geographically, substantive changes in the distribution of patients per 100,000 population had also occurred. Though the West and Southwest remained the focus of states with the lowest ratios, also included in this group were states such as New Hampshire and Rhode Island, which had two of the highest ratios in 1955. On the other hand, states which previously had some of the lower ratios were in the higher categories by 1987. For example, Kansas, which had a ratio of 215:100,000 in 1955—quite low—reduced its ratio to 67:100,000; this was the third highest ratio in the country in 1987. Overall, the geographic pattern of patients-to-population ratios was much more diverse than in previous years. With the exception of low ratios in the Southwest, there were no notable geographic clusters.

Conclusion

The mental health care situation in the United States remains fluid. It is only relatively recently that use of asylums and hospitals as the locations for care has collapsed. The system was radically altered without adequate planning and funding for community alternatives. The mentally ill continue to be unfortunate pawns in the chess game of mental health care. The homeless, many of whom are mentally ill, are becoming an increasing irritant to society. Initial plans in some states for the total destruction of public asylums and hospitals are now being reconsidered. Instead, refurbishment of old facilities and even the building of new facilities are being discussed in some sectors. The geographic pendulum of care for the mentally ill continues to swing. The hope is that its next cycle will provide an adequate support system for the mentally ill.

Index